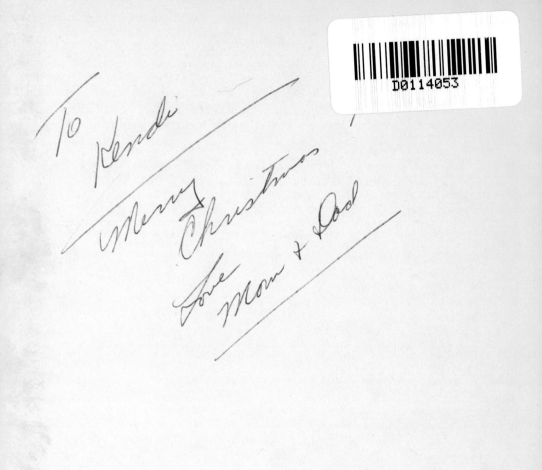

To Kendi

Merry Christmas

Love

Mom & Dad

NO
JOB
FOR A
LADY

ALSO BY M. PHYLLIS LOSE, V.M.D.
Blessed Are the Brood Mares

No Job for a Lady

The Autobiography of
M. Phyllis Lose, V.M.D.
as told to
Daniel Mannix

MACMILLAN PUBLISHING CO., INC.
New York

Macmillan Publishing Co., Inc.
866 Third Avenue, New York, N.Y. 10022
Collier Macmillan Canada, Ltd.

Library of Congress Cataloging in Publication Data
Lose, M   Phyllis.
No job for a lady.
1. Lose, M. Phyllis.   2.   Veterinarians—
Pennsylvania—Biography.   I.   Mannix, Daniel Pratt,
1911–   II.   Title.
SF613.L67A36   630.1'08'90924   [B]   79-14790
ISBN   0-02-575240-5

First Printing 1979

PRINTED IN THE UNITED STATES OF AMERICA

CONTENTS

INTRODUCTION: A FOAL IS BORN, *3*

[1] PONIES AND PROBLEMS, *14*

[2] FIFTEEN-YEAR-OLD PROFESSIONAL, *33*

[3] GIRL MEETS HORSE, *53*

[4] STATE CHAMPIONSHIP, *71*

[5] WOMAN HORSE DOCTOR, *98*

[6] OPERATING IN A BURNING BARN, *115*

[7] I JOIN THE CIRCUS, *129*

[8] CIRCUS HORSES, *150*

[9] WITH THE MOUNTED POLICE, *166*

[10] DISASTERS, *185*

[11] MY OWN HOSPITAL, *208*

NO
JOB
FOR A
LADY

INTRODUCTION:
A FOAL IS BORN

THE BUZZER THAT SIGNALS AN EMERGENCY WENT OFF IN MY ear and I was out of bed and into my boots and coveralls before it had stopped. Mother must have gotten a phone call that something was wrong and was signaling me from her bedroom. The illuminated dial of the electric clock was the only light in the room; it showed the time to be a few minutes after one in the morning. That was to be expected. It was February and the height of the foaling season, and as I specialize in equine obstetrics, this was the busiest time of the year for me. According to the regulations of the National Racing Association, all horses born in the same year are considered to be the same age and compete against each other in events, although naturally it makes a great deal of difference whether a horse was born in the early or the later part of the year. One that is ten or twelve months older has a tremendous advantage; so all breeders try to have their foals born as close to January 1 as possible, which means you are on call day and night. When I first got my veterinary diploma, equine obstetrics was considered too hard work for a woman. It *is* hard work, but the thrill of bringing new life into the world more than makes up for it.

I zipped up my boots and coveralls. All my clothes fasten with zippers to save time, for if a mare is having trouble, seconds count. Just then, I wanted a cup of coffee more than a long life, but there wasn't time. I picked up the interoffice telephone.

3

Mother was at the other end, waiting in her bedroom for me to answer the buzzer. She takes all outside calls because often I'm not home and may have to be contacted on the car radio.

"It's Echo Valley Farm—William Fitler's stables," Mother informed me. Mother is marvelously efficient; she knows all the principal stables and who owns them.

"I know. That chestnut mare of his is in foal. Is she in trouble?"

"Bad trouble. Sounds like a breech delivery. You'd better get there fast. Norma will meet you at the door with a Thermos of coffee. You can drink while you drive."

"God bless Norma," I said, and hung up.

Still half-asleep, I stumbled down the stairs. Sure enough, there was my sister Norma, in bathrobe and slippers, with the Thermos. I grabbed it, muttering, "Thanks. I'm sorry you had to get up."

"That's all right. I haven't an hour's drive over icy roads ahead of me to deliver a mare." She hesitated. "I heard Mr. Fitler over the phone. He's half-crazy with worry."

I could imagine that he would be. Mr. Fitler took a strictly commercial attitude toward his horses. The chestnut mare was valued at $50,000 and the foal's sire was Sporting Chance, whose stud fee was $10,000. Yes, I could understand Mr. Fitler's being worried.

Norma opened the door as I huddled into an overcoat and plunged into the night. The murderous cold took my breath away. The thermometer had been in the low twenties all day; now it was in the low teens. We live in a Colonial house, not far from Valley Forge Park near Philadelphia, and our windows saw Washington and his army march past to fight the Battle of the Clouds 5 miles away. In spite of developments and superhighways, most of the country hasn't changed too much since those days. It is still farming country and horse country. There are a number of the great estates that made the Main Line so famous in its day that when Queen Victoria asked a Philadelphia debutante where she lived, the girl replied in astonishment, "Why, on the Main Line, of course!" Grubbs Mill Road, which runs past our house, goes back even before the time of William Penn to the first Swedish explorers. It's lined by trees, which makes it cool and shaded in summer, and when the ground is covered with snow, the trees help to show you the turns and twists so you don't find yourself in a field surrounded by surprised sheep. Some are old sugar maples with trunks 8 feet in circumference.

The yellow squares of light from the kitchen windows shone on the brown, frozen grass that crunched under my boots as I ran for the garage. A keen wind was blowing and the cold hurt my lungs. Luckily it was a clear night with steel-blue stars and a bone-white moon. My car was in the garage, loaded with everything I might need, which was plenty, for I never know what to expect and have to be ready for any emergency. Unlike the plumber who forgets his tools, if I had to return for anything, my patient might well be dead before I got back. (I drive a Cadillac, the only make of car that can stand up under the treatment I give it.)

In the back of the car was a refrigerator where perishable drugs were kept. When the car was running, the refrigerator ran off the battery, but now it was plugged by a long cable into a wall socket. One of my recurrent nightmares (I have a collection) is forgetting to unplug the connection and driving off with 5 yards of cable dragging behind the car. This time I remembered.

I drove past our pasture surrounded by white post-and-rail that gleamed like a procession of ghosts in the darkness and out the iron gates. Then I turned west on Grubbs Mill Road. As soon as I was clear, I picked up the microphone, said, "KGH, six-five-six," and waited.

That is our code call. Our radio covers a radius of 50 miles and we need a special license to operate it. All our calls are monitored by the government and no conversation except for business purposes is permitted. I say 50 miles, but sometimes through freak conditions we can pick up broadcasts from much further away. Once I called Norma and she reminded me that I hadn't eaten for twenty-four hours. "You'll find a sandwich in the refrigerator among the drugs," she added. I told her that I didn't have time to stop. A man's voice broke in, "Eat that sandwich, damn it, and stop at the first place you can and get some coffee!" I asked, astonished, "Who are you?" "This is the Ohio Highway Patrol and we're saving your local police the trouble of scraping you off some tree."

Now I heard Norma's voice. "Mr. Fitler called again. The mare is growing violent. He wants to know if you've left yet."

I'd been hoping for some reassuring news, such as, "You can take it a little easy. Both front feet are out." In spite of the ice-covered, twisting road, I stepped up speed. At the same time, I managed to get the top off the Thermos and gulp a mouthful of the almost boiling coffee. One of the several skills I've had to develop is learning how to drink and drive.

There would be no sleep for any of us that night. Norma would stay up with the receiver in her hand waiting for a call from me in case anything went wrong. Mother would be at the telephone, keeping touch with the Fitlers or, in case there was a second emergency call, relaying it to another veterinarian who was available.

These car-broadcasting units are a godsend. I know some veterinarians who use a beeper tied to their belts that gives off a buzzing sound when their office wants to call them. It has the advantage that even if they are in a stable or a field they can be alerted, but I don't use them. It generally takes too long to find a phone after the beeper goes off so you can call back and find out what's happened.

I left Grubbs Mill Road and turned onto a modern highway, running straight across country. Now the friendly trees were gone, their place taken by high-tension lines, overpasses for the new turnpikes, and lines of industrial complexes that had fled the high tax rate of Philadelphia for the suburbs. At this time of night there was no traffic and I pressed down the accelerator. Then the radio squawked and I heard Norma's voice saying anxiously, "Hurry! He doesn't think the mare can last much longer."

From long experience I could picture the tortured animal, half-crazy with pain, thrashing on the straw, the foal kicking and struggling inside of her, both growing steadily weaker until one or both died. It was a sickening picture, but now I was only a few miles from the Fitler farm. I had left the industrial complexes behind and was in open farm country, except for an occasional tree and the upsweeping girders of the tension line towers that showed against the night sky like the skeletons of marching giants. I increased my speed. Suddenly there was a report like a gunshot, the car swerved wildly back and forth across the road while I fought the wheel. Then I skated to a stop. A rear tire had blown.

This was a disaster. The car had been overloaded and I knew it. Norma and I had a running feud over how much should be put in the trunk. From time to time I would get mad, especially when the back was so full of instruments, drugs, buckets, trays, and bottles that I couldn't find what I was looking for. Then I'd get Norma to take most of the stuff out, ignoring her protests. Sure enough, a few days later I'd be off on a job and couldn't find something I vitally needed. Then, according to Norma, I'd call her and complain that she'd taken it out of the car without telling me. So Norma would put everything back in again and the overloaded car would break a spring on some rutty back road. This time, though, I'd really done it. Well, thank heaven the radio was working.

I lifted the mike and called, "KGH, six-five-six Emergency! Emergency!" and waited for the familiar reply.

There was no answer. I tried again. Again no answer. I swore, which is something I don't often do, and tried a third time. I couldn't believe it but the radio was dead—utterly, completely dead. Here I was on a lonely road at two in the morning with two animals dying a few miles away.

But the radio couldn't be dead; it had been working perfectly well only a few minutes before. Perhaps the antenna had come loose. I got out to check it, feeling, for one of the very few times in my life, close to hysterics. The intense cold that fastened on me as I got out of the car brought me around.

I looked up at the antenna and saw at once what the trouble was. The antenna was all right, but by a miracle of bad luck I had come to stop under a power line that crossed the road at this point. The radio wouldn't function under a power line.

It was bad but not a total disaster, as I could run on the rim for the few remaining miles to the stables. It might ruin the car but I could save the mare and her foal. Certainly I could get out from under that power line. I got back in, put the car in gear, and pressed down on the accelerator.

In the rear-view mirror I saw a shower of sparks where the metal rim spun on the macadam. The car was anchored to the road and, what was even worse, the sparks were showering in a fountain of fire on my gas tank. I switched off the motor fast and tried to think.

I knew the road and it was a lonely one. There was almost no chance of anyone going by until dawn. I got out again and looked around. Nothing but fields and woods on every hand. Not a sign of a house. I could imagine the sufferings of the mare; probably the foal was dead by now. Norma would try calling me in a while, and when I didn't respond, she'd eventually call the police and they'd find me. By that time, the mare as well as the foal would almost surely be dead.

Then, far away over the fields, I saw a pinhole of light no bigger than a firefly. I shifted my position, blinked my eyes, and looked again until I was sure. There must be a house out there and someone was still up.

The field was fenced with several strands of barbed wire; no elegant (and easily climbable) post-and-rail for these farmers. I had a pretty good idea that I'd encounter a number of these fences before I made it to the house, so I left my coat in the car and started out over the frozen ground. Some years before I'd tried climbing barbed-wire fences in an overcoat and I'd rather freeze than try it again.

It had looked a long way to the farmhouse but that was an optical illusion; it was twice as far. The old farmhouses were built only a few feet from the roads so the inhabitants didn't have far to shovel their way out after a snowstorm, but that, of course, was before the days of heavy traffic and motorized vehicles with their noise and smell. Today, farmers want to get as far away from roads as possible, and I don't blame them except when it's the middle of the night and I'm falling into ditches and struggling over fences. Still, the light kept growing larger and brighter until I finally was able to make out the shape of the house against the night sky. The light was in what I suppose you'd call the living room and I saw four men sitting around a table playing cards. They all seemed to be smoking so the room was somewhat foggy and there were so many beer cans on the table I don't see how they found room for the cards.

I staggered up the steps onto the porch and pounded on the door. There had been a murmur of voices and an occasional laugh. Now there was sudden silence. I beat on the door again and shouted. Finally it was opened by a big man wearing overalls. He stared at me unbelievingly.

"I'm a veterinarian, answering an emergency call," I explained. "My car's broken down. May I use your phone?"

The four men continued to look at me as though I were a ghost. At last, the man in the overalls asked, "What did you say you were?"

"A veterinarian. A vet." As they still looked blank I said desperately, "A horse doctor. A mare's having trouble foaling and I have to get in touch with my office."

I should explain that at that time—the 1950s—there were only two women veterinarians in Pennsylvania and they worked only with small animals. To these farmers, the idea of a woman vet was incredible. One of the men at the table who was enormously fat and wore a leather jacket said kindly, "You mean you want us to call a vet for your sick horse?"

The fact that I'm small, slender, and blond didn't do me any good either in impressing these old-time farmers. "I am a doctor," I told him, fighting to control my temper. "Look at my coveralls. My car's out on the road, full of instruments and medicines. Do you want to take a look at it?"

"Now you'd better have a drink," suggested another farmer, leaning back and getting a can of beer off a wardrobe. "Just where is this sick horse?"

I finally managed to persuade them to let me use their telephone. "Where are you?" Norma half-shouted, as soon as she heard my voice. "Mr. Fitler's been calling again. The mare's weakening rapidly. I couldn't get you on the radio. What's happened?"

I explained briefly and asked for the Fitlers' number. Then I called the stable. One of the grooms answered, but as soon as he heard my name, he summoned Mr. Fitler.

Mr. Fitler was half out of his head. He said the mare was all but dead; he'd given up hope of the foal.

I told him where my car was. "Send someone for me as quickly as you can," I told him. "I'll take what I think I'll need from the car. I'll be there waiting so don't waste any time."

I thanked my hosts, who had finally decided that I wasn't

insane, and said goodbye. Now that I knew the way across the fields, it was easier going back. At the car, I got out several stainless-steel pails, syringes, medicines, polyethylene sleeves, my obstetric box, and the instruments I thought I might need. I had barely finished when a car shot up beside me and stopped, peeling rubber as the brakes screamed.

Mrs. Fitler was driving. Luckily, it was a station wagon. I put my pails and instruments in the rear, then climbed into the front seat beside her. I'm used to fast driving in an emergency, but the way Mrs. Fitler drove frankly terrified me. She kept telling me about the mare, what a valuable animal it was and how much they had counted on the foal. Occasionally she'd burst into tears. Thank heaven the ride was short and we didn't meet any other cars.

The Fitler farm was a huge estate of over 150 acres. There were two hundred mares on it during the breeding season and five stallions. Even during the off season, there were never less than a hundred mares. There were three barns: the original bank barn was over two hundred years old. Like most barns of that period, it had been built into the side of a hill to make it easier for the teams to drag the hay wagons into the vast loft. In the lower part were the stalls: the hill kept this cool in summer and sheltered it from high winds in winter.

We drove past fields now bare and empty but in summer brilliant with growing oats or alfalfa, clover and timothy, ready to be turned into hay. As we reached the bank barn, the double door of a box stall flew open and a gust of steam came from the hot interior. There was Mr. Fitler, flanked by grooms, standing in the doorway. He was smoking a cigar and waving me in. As I got out of the car, he shouted: "Where the hell have you been? The mare's just gone down. We tried to keep her up and walking but it was too damned hard. That foal's worth a quarter of a million to me!"

One of the tragedies—and to anyone fond of horses it is a real tragedy—of working with thoroughbreds is that they are often so valuable that monetary considerations wipe out all other factors. Every other physical, and mental, trait is sacrificed for speed. As the result of intensive breeding, only too often the animal is so delicate that he or she cannot live a normal life. Further, the owner has frequently invested so much money in that animal that even a minor injury which slows the racer down can be a crippling blow to his bank account. Under such circumstances, working with horses is no longer fun; there is no real affection between the master and the mount. It is all a grim business of profit.

Toting my obstetric box, I went into the stall. There were six or seven men—grooms and stable boys—grouped around the recumbent body of the mare. Her eyes were rolled back so you could see the whites; she was shaking and gasping, obviously in terrible pain. There was no sign of the foal but her placental water had already broken—her hind legs and the straw around her were soaked with it.

I had to relieve the pain first before I could do anything with the tortured animal. I gave her an injection to sedate her, and while it was taking effect sent one of the men with two of my stainless-steel buckets for hot water. Meanwhile, I had another man bandage her tail to keep the dirty hairs from infecting her perineal region. As soon as the water arrived, I washed out her vulva and slipped a polyethylene sleeve over my hand.

The mare was quiet now, only semi-conscious, and not suffering greatly. I slowly worked my hand deeper and deeper inside until I could touch the foal. The men had been shouting at each other but now they were still, except for Mr. Fitler, who kept marching up and down, chewing on his cigar.

The instant I touched the foal, I had an awful feeling it was dead. There was no "tone" to the little body. It was soggy and inert like a piece of butcher's meat. I put my finger in the mouth —I could feel no tongue reflex. I felt the eye. Did I imagine it or was there a faint response? Yet I could feel no pulse and no heartbeat.

Lying on the straw with my arm in the unhappy mare, I wondered whether, if I'd been more careful about overloading the car, I might have arrived in time. I would have to tell Mr. Fitler that his foal was dead. I was too tired and discouraged to worry about the outburst of fury that would follow; I only wished I could have saved the poor little animal.

"I hate to tell you this," I said at last. "I'm sorry, but I think the foal is dead."

He stopped his pacing. "How can you tell?" he shouted.

"I'm not positive but I can feel no real signs of life. We'll have to worry about the mare. She's very weak and sinking fast."

He resumed his pacing, his handsome face flushed. "A ten-thousand-dollar stud fee wasted! A year's expenses keeping her gone down the drain. Now I won't be able to breed that mare for another year—more waste. Why couldn't you have gotten here sooner?" He strode up and down, cursing.

Meanwhile, I was getting ready to extract the foal. It wasn't a job I liked. The legs of a foal are tremendously long and getting them in the correct position for delivery is difficult. Any mistake, and the lining of the uterus could easily be torn. That meant the mare would never foal again, even if she lived, which would be unlikely. Or the foal might be hopelessly lodged inside her. I had heard of such cases. Then the fetus had to be cut up inside the mother with a wire saw and taken out bit by bit—a grisly and dangerous procedure. Yet time was important. The mother might begin to hemorrhage, develop septicemia (bacteria in the bloodstream), or die of shock; on the other hand, if the foal were pulled out too abruptly, the reproductive tract might be permanently destroyed.

My greatest concern was that the placental fluid had been lost and the little body was dry. There was nothing to lubricate its passage through the uterus, and under these conditions the lining of the wall would almost certainly tear. That would be fatal.

Fortunately, I had brought a stomach pump with me and several gallons of medical mineral oil. I pumped the oil into the mare's uterus. After a little time, I was able to insert my hand and reposition the foal, but try as I would the forelegs remained locked in a twisted position. Slowly, inch by inch, I worked the legs out. Suddenly the almost unconscious mother gave a heave and the foal slid out into my arms, knocking me over. Once on the straw, he lay motionless, the eyes staring, seemingly lifeless. I wiped the oil from his mouth and blew into his lungs; at the same time, I kneaded the little body, trying to make him breathe. All at once I saw one of the eyes move and the foal sucked in air. Incredibly, he was alive. Now I was able to untwist the forelegs, and in a few minutes, the foal staggered to his feet.

Mr. Fitler stared at the foal as though he were seeing a miracle. "Will he be all right?" he asked, after a time.

"I think so, but first I'll have to get the mare up so he can nurse." A mare's first milk contains certain ingredients vitally important to the foal. I started running fluids into the mare's veins to replace the loss of electrolytes during the stress period; these are minute particles of chemical matter in the bloodstream that are crucial to an animal's well-being. In an hour the mare was on her feet and the little foal reeled uncertainly on his long, stiltlike legs to nurse.

In this case I was lucky in being able to relax and reposition the forelegs for proper presentation. Sometimes their joints are hopelessly locked in such a way that they cannot be released. Then, even if the foal is born alive, it must be put to sleep as it could never walk. We don't know what causes this condition; it may be inherited or congenital. It is not the result of an accident, as far as we can tell. It seems to turn up more frequently in certain families of thoroughbreds—unfortunately, frequently the fastest. I suspect it is the fault of the breeders who aren't careful enough about bloodlines. Breeders of thoroughbreds want to produce an animal that can run away from its own tail. To get speed, they'll sacrifice every other consideration, including the horse's health.

At first the mother seemed almost frightened of the strange creature that had caused her so much suffering. But I did not leave until I saw her begin to lick him. I knew then that everything would be all right. I'm glad to say the mare recovered very well and the little colt eventually distinguished himself on the track, although I nearly lost both of them that night. Shortly afterwards, the Fitlers moved away and gave up horse breeding. Perhaps it was just as well.

I

PONIES AND PROBLEMS

As long as I can remember, I've always loved animals—
especially horses. When I was three years old, I got lost following
a bread wagon horse with the loveliest brass-studded harness
(yes, in the 1920s there were still horses pulling wagons in Philadelphia). Mother spent two hours searching the streets of
Springfield—a suburb of Philadelphia where we lived—and
when she finally found me, she didn't know whether to cry with
relief or murder me. She compromised by making me wheel my
little sister around in her baby carriage whenever I went out,
thinking that would slow me down. She was wrong. The next day
when suppertime came, we were missing. After a little thought,
Mother knew where to look: she went to the nearest blacksmith's
forge. Sure enough, there were baby Shirley and I watching
round-eyed the marvelous shoeing of the great draft horses that
pulled the Abbott Dairy milk wagons. On Sunday afternoons,
when Father drove us around in his elderly convertible, I was
strictly forbidden to stand up in the back seat. I always obeyed—
unless we passed a mounted policeman. Then, in spite of everything, I was hanging out of the car as long as that magnificent
charger was in sight.

Actually, I came by my love of horses naturally enough. My
parents were of Pennsylvania Dutch stock and came from Montour County in the north-central part of the state, where for

many years they had owned and operated a horse and cattle farm. We still own it, although now, alas, the horses have been replaced by tractors. It is near the little town of Exchange—so called because in the old days the stagecoaches used to exchange horses there. It produces some of the best corn, buckwheat, soybeans, and clover hay I've ever seen, and Mother drives up there twice a month to talk with the farmer and see how things are going. One of my favorite horses is buried there with all her tack and I often go up to sit by her grave and think of the good times we had together.

I don't know when I first began to dream of being an equine veterinarian, but I always wanted to do something that would keep me working with horses. In those days, the idea of a woman being a "horse doctor" was virtually unthinkable, although Mother sympathized with me. As a girl, she had ridden all the horses on the farm, except the high-tempered stallion, even though it was not much fun as they were all draft horses. Mother was always adventurous. Even after she married Father, moved away from Montour, and settled down in the outskirts of Philadelphia, she still was ready to try anything—or have us try. Father was the practical member of the family. He was also of Pennsylvania Dutch extraction, a tall man slightly under 6 feet, who because he loved to eat and enjoy life always had a weight problem. As a young man he had realized early that the life of a farmer was hard work with little reward; opportunity lay in the cities. So he went into the poultry business, bringing down truckloads of chickens, ducks, turkeys, and guinea fowl from the upcountry farms to Philadelphia. When I was seven, in the early 1930s, a boy cousin and I used to go with him. Our job was to arrange the coops in the back of the truck and feed and water the birds. It was quite a responsibility. If the coops were stacked incorrectly, the birds would suffocate, and if we neglected a coop, they would die of thirst. Father would take the poultry to the best hotels and restaurants first, let them have their pick, for which they paid him a premium, then unload the rest of the birds on the downtown market. We each got $1.50 a week, of which I would squander a nickel for an ice cream cone. The rest I saved, hoping someday to buy a horse.

As a child, I always seemed to be busy. I don't mean by this that I was overworked; I loved the feeling of responsibility and the fact that Father trusted my judgment with the birds. Of course, I liked being able to earn money. I feel sorry for children today who complain that they have nothing to do. I realize that with everything so mechanized, there aren't the opportunities for small jobs that there were then. Still, it's too bad and must be frustrating for modern youngsters.

Although he did not ride, Father loved horses and used to take all of us to horse shows in the neighborhood and also to the races. I don't remember his ever betting but he liked to guess the winners. He was pretty good at it, for he knew horses well. In the evenings, we would have a family musicale. All of the family were musically inclined, especially Father, who made money on the side tuning organs. He played the piano in our impromptu sessions and we all played some instrument. Mine was the violin and I know that Mother hoped someday I would be a violinist. I enjoyed playing, but it wasn't anything like horses.

In Springfield, we lived in a center hall Colonial on a corner lot with an acre of land that seemed enormous to us children. We had a garden, a lawn that had to be kept mowed, and several big trees perfect for climbing. We also had a little black and white dog named Snappy and we amused ourselves teaching him tricks. Snappy was the nicest dog I've ever known; he had a real personality and was very affectionate. He stayed with Mother while we were at school, but as soon as it was time for us to come home, he would desert her and be at the front door, waiting for us. He was my first pet.

When we were little children, Mother always put us to sleep with horse stories of the old days on the farm and sometimes Father would come up and add his reminiscences. When I was ten, I decided that life wasn't worth living without a pony. I had saved up the huge sum of $25, which I thought was plenty for a horse. There was some extra room in our garage and I set about building a stall there. It wasn't much of a stall and wouldn't have held a really athletic guinea pig; but I considered it a masterpiece. I even invited some neighborhood children in to admire it. The next day, I got my first real blow. A little boy told me, "My father says you can't keep a horse here. The zoning regulations won't let you."

I had never heard of zoning regulations. I dashed to the house to ask Mother. She was away shopping and Father, of course, was working. I had dreamed so long of owning a pony that I couldn't believe all those long hours I had spent loading chicken coops, building the stall, and earning my money had been wasted. I had counted so much on getting a pony that I had even gone to the local hay and feed store to price hay and grain. I had decided that by working all my summer vacation and after school in the winter, I could just support a pony. Now it seemed that horses weren't allowed to be kept in private homes in Springfield. I felt as though the end of the world had come and there was nothing left to live for.

Like all the children I knew, I had unbounded trust in the police. Policemen were kindly men, all-powerful, who used their power only to help other people, especially children. I got on my bike and rode down to the local police station. I remember how the desk sergeant stared at me when I walked in.

"Please, is there any law that says I can't keep a pony in our garage?" I asked.

The sergeant sat looking at me for quite some time. I couldn't imagine why he didn't answer me. I didn't realize that my face was streaked with tears, my skinny little legs were trembling, and my voice shook. After a long while, the sergeant said, "There's no reason why you can't, as long as you keep him clean so he isn't a health hazard."

"Oh, thank you, thank you!" I cried, and raced home on my bike. Mother had returned and I told her the good news. She looked at me gravely and asked, "Does having a horse mean that much to you, Phyllis?"

I could only look at her. It was such a strange question.

That evening, Mother and Father had a conference. After it was over, they called me in. "If we get a pony, Phyllis, you know it can't be just for you. All the children would have to share it."

That was quite all right with me. There were four of us· Norma, the oldest, then me, Shirley, and Lloyd, the only boy. Today we hear a great deal about "sibling rivalry," and I won't say we never disagreed, but generally we got along well together and shared everything. Part of the reason was that we all had our

17

own interests and were too occupied with our different affairs to quarrel. Besides, I was so delighted at the prospect of getting a pony that I didn't care about anything else.

Father knew of a reliable horse dealer in the northeast part of the city on Roosevelt Boulevard, which was then nearly all farming country. We all drove up there together in the family car, the other children nearly as crazy with excitement as I was. The dealer had a stable and several horses and ponies. I believe he made part of his living by giving children pony rides. One pony, a pinto, was for sale. He was rather large for a pony—14½ hands*—and rather old, so the dealer was willing to let him go fairly cheaply. Father had him vanned back to Springfield and he was installed in his new home in the garage, although first Father made a number of repairs to my makeshift stall.

The pony's name was Flash, and we all thought that he was the most wonderful thing in the world. Although we shared him, it was my special responsibility to keep his stall mucked out. I remembered what the police sergeant had told me and was terrified that Flash would be taken away from us if he wasn't kept spotlessly clean. The tiniest bit of dung was promptly whisked away, he got clean straw every morning, and I sprinkled lime on the floor to make sure there was no odor.

I suspect that this was the beginning of my mania for cleanliness and sterilization, which has since nearly driven my friends and family crazy. Even I know that I carry it to ridiculous lengths. I suppose in the back of my mind is always the fear that unless everything is antiseptically clean, I'll lose Flash. I'm still boiling and scrubbing and disinfecting everything I use far more than is necessary.

In spite of all my hard work, I made a mess of things, especially by modern standards. Of course, I used straw for bedding —everyone did then. Straw was cheap and easy to obtain. Now it is expensive and hard to get, which is just as well, for it makes a poor bedding. It contains antigens—substances that irritate the lining of the lungs and produce heaves, somewhat like asthma in a human being. Heaves were one of the commonest of horse ailments in the old days; now they are occurring less and less.

* A hand is 4 inches (14½ hands is the limit for ponies).

Today, bedding is usually composed of shavings, peatmoss, or the commercial Staz-drie, although I think the best is Astroturf. It is springy and cushions the animal's weight. It can be graded for better drainage and is easily washed. Luckily, through our farm we had access to the best wheat straw, which contains few antigens, so I made out fairly well.

Then there was the floor. At first, I used boards laid a little apart to allow for drainage. But Father, with a great deal of effort, installed a clay floor, which was considered the last word in superior flooring at the time. Now we know that clay harbors fungoid and bacterial infections. Fortunately, I used plenty of lime, although today I would have used a Betadine solution that is far better. My parents showed me how to remove the straw bedding for a couple hours each day to allow for circulation of air to dry out the clay.

We children spoiled Flash, which was a mistake. He got fed far too much. The standard hay for horses in those days was timothy, but Father felt that there wasn't enough nourishment in it for a large horse, worked hard, and he was right. We had the farm to draw on for legumes—alfalfa, clover, and soybean—which were called "cow hay" and considered too good for horses. I still think the legumes are the best hay going, if you can get them. When you do, they usually run around $150 a ton and few people can afford them. We fed Flash all the legumes he could eat.

We quickly found that even a pony requires quite a lot of tack; what might be called his "outfit." Father supplied us with a saddle and bridle (those cost too much for us), but we kids chipped in to buy the rest. That included a halter, a blanket, a cooler (a light, openwork sheet to put on a horse when he is overheated), a curry comb, hoof pick, brushes, a sweat scraper, and buckets. Keeping a horse was expensive.

But Flash was worth it. He had a real personality. He would whinny whenever he heard us coming and seemed to enjoy being ridden. We taught him various tricks such as bowing, counting (pawing a number of times with one foot), rearing on command, and so on. Mother showed us how to do it. If you said, "Bow!" and put a piece of carrot on the ground, Flash would bend over to get it. After a while whenever you said, "Bow!" he'd bend his

19

head to look for the carrot. Of course, you always gave him a piece as a reward. If you tapped his foot lightly with a whip, he'd paw the ground. Then he learned to paw on cue when you pointed with the whip. You could ask him how much were four and four and he would start pawing. When he reached eight, you'd lower the whip. To make him rear, you'd run in on him and wave your hands. After a few times, whenever you raised your hands, he'd rear.

I remember once when I went into his stall, I spoke to him in a funny voice as a joke. To my surprise, he came over and put his head on my shoulder; I still can't imagine why. From then on, whenever I spoke in that special way, he'd run to me and put his cheek against mine. It became his most popular trick.

There is also a lot of work connected with a pony. They have to be groomed daily. There's an old saying, "A good grooming is equivalent to a good meal," meaning a horse gets as much value out of a grooming as out of food. Grooming with a curry comb and brush removes loose hair, stimulates the coat, and gives the animal a sense of well-being. Like most living creatures, horses like to be fussed over. The old-time grooms had a special way of hissing through their teeth when they curried a horse. They were confident that it soothed the animal. Perhaps it did, but as far as I know it is now a lost art.

We didn't have Flash shod because we rode him only over soft ground. Every couple of months, Father would run a rasp over his hoofs to keep them from getting too long and to smooth out any cracks. For some reason or other, we had trouble getting a blacksmith in Springfield, but with Father's help, we really didn't need one. We were careful to keep Flash's little hoofs cleaned out with a pick to prevent thrush. This is a fungus that forms in the frog of the hoof and usually is the result of neglect, especially letting the horse stand in a dirty stall. I always kept Flash's stall immaculate. Even so, it was a good idea to make sure the over-growth of the hoofs was trimmed and cleaned out every day.

For six months, Flash was the perfect pony. Then he began to change. We couldn't believe the way he acted toward us. First, he wouldn't let us put the tack (saddle and bridle) on him, although previously he had always seemed delighted to go for a ride. Then we couldn't even get into the stall with him; he would put his ears back, show his teeth, and actually attack us. We tried everything we could think of to win him back, bringing him all his favorite tidbits like carrots and apples and giving him extra feedings of grain (like all ponies, Flash was a regular pig), but he grew meaner and meaner. Out of loyalty to him, we didn't tell Father and Mother about the change. Then one afternoon Mother was looking out the window and saw all four of us running out of Flash's stall with Flash chasing us with bared teeth. That evening, she told Father. He went to the garage himself to see if it were true and a few minutes later we saw Father running for his life with Flash after him. To tell the truth, once Flash had shown you who was boss, he would stop, and I don't believe he would have really hurt anyone; but he certainly put up a wonderful bluff.

Father's verdict was: "That pony will have to go before he hurts someone."

Mother agreed, but on being confronted by four sobbing children, our parents relented a little. At last, Father offered a compromise. He would take Flash to the Four Horsemen Riding Club and see if they could do anything with him. The Four Horsemen was only 2 miles away and was a private boarding stable, quite elegant. There was an indoor riding hall big enough for horse shows to be held there, and it was located on the edge of some woods laced with bridle paths that ran for miles. The owner was Armor MacClay, a dignified older man with white hair who always dressed immaculately and looked exactly what he was, a highly competent gentleman rider. We children had only seen him from a distance but we stood in awe of him. Although we knew that Mr. MacClay had a great reputation as an expert on horses, we were still reluctant to entrust our precious Flash to him. Mr. MacClay might not understand what a sensitive creature Flash really was and be mean to him, especially if Flash tried to bite him; however, it was either that or losing Flash altogether.

Father contributed one of his poultry trucks for a horse van. It took the combined efforts of the whole family to load Flash, and even then we couldn't have done it if Father hadn't used a nose twitch. This is a loop of soft cord fastened to the end of a short stick; the loop is slipped over the horse's nose (a very delicate part of his anatomy), and then the cord is twisted. It takes a most determined horse to fight against a nose twitch.

We drove to the Four Horsemen and after unloading Flash (which was a great deal easier than loading him), stood around in an anxious circle while Mr. MacClay examined him.

"What have you been feeding him?" Mr. MacClay demanded.

"Well, he gets all the legume hay he can eat," I explained. "Then I give him a bucket of sweetfeed in the morning and another at night."

"I give him a bucket of whole oats. He likes them better than the sweetfeed," Norma put in.

"And I make sure he gets plenty of corn," added Lloyd.

"I'm the one who brings him his hot mash," said Shirley proudly.

"Why has he gotten so aggressive?" asked Mother anxiously.

"Why hasn't he foundered, you mean," snapped Mr. Mac-Clay. "Now see here, children, a pony should never be given any grain at all, except perhaps a small handful as a treat. And nothing but timothy hay."

"But there's not much nourishment in timothy!" Father exclaimed.

"That's why I recommend it. That little monster is as fat as a brood sow. No wonder you can't do anything with him! Leave him here a couple of weeks and he'll be a different pony."

"You're not going to hurt him or starve him, are you?" whimpered Shirley.

Mr. MacClay whirled on her. "Little girl, I never abused a horse in my life and I won't have a man on the place who ill treats an animal. But there's a difference between cruelty and discipline, and if you're going to work with horses, you must understand the difference. In the first place, any grain-fed pony will become incorrigible. That's basic. Secondly, a horse must always realize that you are the master, not him. A horse that insists on doing what he wants to do is no use to anyone and will end up at the knackers. Now that's what I call being really cruel to him."

So we left Flash at the Four Horsemen. I rode my bike over every afternoon to see how he was coming along. It took only a few days to see an improvement in Flash's disposition. He was put on a strict diet and exercised by a man who would put up with no nonsense. If Flash went at anyone with his ears laid back and his teeth showing, he got a rap on his nose that discouraged him. In fact, he did so well there that Father decided to board him permanently at the Four Horsemen.

I never forgot that lesson. Anyone working with horses must learn the difference between cruelty and discipline. Especially for children, it is often a hard distinction to make. Horses respect discipline but they resent cruelty and will turn on you. Discipline is not so much punishment as it is keeping the horse under control. Then, too, you must understand horses. If a horse has been locked up in a stall for a couple of days, you can't expect to tack him up and start riding him at once; he will be too restless. This is not viciousness, and if you try to punish him when he starts to buck and kick up his heels, he will resent it. Let him have a short run in the paddock to get the kinks out of him and he'll be all right. Personally, I've found that the best form of control—when control is needed—is the nose twitch. With the twitch, you don't hurt the horse; he hurts himself if he fights it and he soon comes to realize that.

I spent a great deal of time at the Four Horsemen after that. The horses were beautifully taken care of. I remember especially the huge cookers where the mash was prepared. They were going from ten in the morning until five in the afternoon. The mash was composed of whole oats, a small percentage of corn and wheat bran, and served warm to the horses. I believe it was the perfect diet when supplemented with good hay. Today, no one would go to the expense or trouble of cooking mash. Horses are usually fed pellets, which are not nearly as good. For one thing, you can never be sure what has gone into the manufacturing of the pellets, and some companies will use inferior grain. About the only advantage to them is that they keep down the dust that hurts a horse's lungs.

I knew my parents couldn't afford riding lessons so I never asked for them and instead spent long hours watching Mr. Mac-Clay and the other riding masters showing people how to ride. I tried not to make a nuisance of myself, but I was always at the edge of the ring listening to the instructions and seeing how it was done. Then Flash and I would go off by ourselves and practice.

Like most youngsters, my ambition was to take a horse over jumps. Following the example Mr. MacClay set with his green jumpers, I laid out a line of trotting poles on the ground parallel to each other. Then, with Flash on a lunge line, I led him across them. A lunge is a 35-foot line made of webbing that fastens onto the horse's halter. The poles were spaced so that Flash could trot over them easily. This got him accustomed to going over obstacles and also taught him to maintain a set pace. After several weeks, I was able to raise the trotting poles a few inches above the ground. Then, still keeping Flash on the lunge line, I took him over small jumps. When I finally mounted him, I was careful always to maintain the same speed as I came into the jump and to approach it at the center at right angles. When actually jumping, I let Flash have his head. A horse focuses on distant objects by raising his head; for nearer objects, he lowers it. So when coming into a jump, he has to be able to move his head readily. As he comes into the jump holding his head high, he can't look directly down because his muzzle is too wide: he must be free to choose his own head position.

Flash learned to like jumping; or, to be more accurate, he liked to please me and would try to take any jump I put him at. My first great triumph was when I asked Mr. MacClay what he thought was the highest jump Flash could take.

"A little fellow like that couldn't possibly jump more than three feet six," he assured me.

"I have him jumping four feet already," I told him.

Mr. MacClay smiled and shook his head. "It's impossible."

I tacked up Flash and took him over three 4-foot jumps while Mr. MacClay watched. He got a stick and measured the jumps himself. "I still don't believe it," he said, as he straightened up. I was so proud of Flash I tried him at even bigger jumps, but 4 feet proved to be his limit.

Although Mother no longer rode, she knew quite a lot about horses, so I always followed her advice, or rather orders, for Mother was old-fashioned enough to think children should do as they were told. Winter had come but I went to the Four Horsemen every day after school, first stopping at home to leave my books and change my clothes. It rained hard one day and was quite warm, then with the changeableness of Philadelphia weather, there was a hard freeze. When I got home that afternoon, Mother told me, "Don't jump Flash today. It's too slippery."

I promised I wouldn't and went on to the Four Horsemen. I tacked up Flash and we rode around the outside fields a few times. Everything was going smoothly and Flash, thinking that we were going to practice jumping as usual, headed into a post-and-rail jump. I was so intent on guiding him that I forgot what Mother had told me. Just as he made his approach, I heard Mother's voice say distinctly, "Don't jump!" It wasn't my imagination! I heard it as clearly as though she had been standing beside me. It was too late to turn away and Flash rose in the air. As he did so, I felt one of his hind legs slip. For the first time he failed to clear the top rail, tripped, and we both fell heavily. My first thought naturally was Flash, and I examined him carefully. He was all right, but I had fallen on my face. When we got back to the stable, I looked at myself in a mirror. I had a nose the size of a small potato.

When I got home, Mother was working in the kitchen and asked me how everything had gone. "Oh, just splendidly!" I said gaily as I ran past her, taking care to keep my head turned. As soon as I got up to my room, I put cold compresses on my nose and did everything I could think of to shrink it. But nothing did any good. When I came down to supper, there was no hiding it. The whole family stared at me.

"Phyllis, did you jump Flash and fall off?" Mother demanded sternly.

"Yes, I did. I didn't mean to. We just went into the jump by accident."

Father asked quietly, "Is that really true, Phyllis?"

"Yes, it is. And at the last moment I heard Mother telling me not to jump, but it was too late then."

I don't recall Father ever disciplining us. He left that to Mother, even though he always backed her up. Mother always punished us when we were disobedient and I waited miserably to know what my fate would be.

To my surprise, Mother only said, "Don't let it happen again." It never did.

That spring Father got us another pony named Toots and a little cart. When the weather grew warmer, we would go out for picnic suppers along the Wissahickon Creek. In those days— 1937—there was comparatively little traffic and plenty of dirt roads where the cars seldom ventured. We'd put a wickerwork basket full of food that Mother had prepared for us in the back of the cart and drive off, one of us riding Flash. When we found a good place by the creek, we'd stop and have a feast, making sure that Toots and Flash got their share. Toots was a gentle little thing, perfect for driving, but without much personality. I greatly preferred Flash even though he could be a problem at times.

In 1939, I was riding Flash along a bridle trail and decided to take a shortcut home through a district where I'd never been before. Even in those days, the city was beginning to throw out tentacles through the suburbs and the farmers were being pushed out. I passed a farmhouse with a deserted barn. I've always been interested in barns, so I reined in Flash while I looked it over. For some time now I'd been conscious that keeping two ponies at the Four Horsemen had been expensive for Father, and as he'd gotten another car, there was no longer room in our garage even for Flash. I was only about 4 miles from home and this barn looked perfect.

I rode over and examined it. There were no stalls but it would not be too difficult to put some in. There was a huge loft where hay, straw, and feed could be stored. There was running water although no electricity. A 10-acre field surrounded the building, which would make a good exercise ground. Not only could we keep Flash and Toots there but we could also take on boarders and perhaps even make a little money.

Full of my great idea, I rode back to the Four Horsemen, stabled Flash, and then biked home. Mother, as usual, was tolerant. Father was more doubtful and said everything would depend on the rent. The next Saturday, he drove us all over to examine the place; it must have been nearly two hundred years old. The owners were city people who had bought it from a farm family who had been forced to move further out into the country. They had no use for the barn and let us rent it quite cheaply.

We were a busy family for the next six weeks or so. We installed seven box stalls, rigged up a feed bin, built a chute to the loft, painted the walls white and the stalls red. Then we mowed the field (I got one of the men at the Four Horsemen who had a mower to do it), erected a post-and-rail fence, and built some jumps. I knew four or five people who had horses and didn't want to pay the comparatively high rates at the Four Horsemen, so we had no trouble filling the empty stalls. We charged $30 a month board, which included exercising. I like to think that we showed a little profit, but looking back, I don't believe we did more than break even.

As our boarders were constantly changing, I began to learn a little about horse ailments. Some would have a gravel. This was generally caused by stepping on a nail or a sharp stone; the bruise or cut would close over but the infection remained on the inside, so it had to be opened, allowed to drain, and then packed with an antiseptic. Some of the older horses, often ones used in fox hunting, had sidebone. This was a foot unsoundness usually produced by pounding on a hard surface. I now feel that many horses are being bred with feet that are too small and make them susceptible to sidebone. Small feet tend to look well and make a horse fast, but they can't support his weight. I also learned that all horses should have their teeth floated at least once a year. This is done by filing down the sharp edges formed on the upper outside and on the lower inside edges of the teeth. As a horse chews with a lateral motion, he can't digest his food properly if the dental arcade is locked and unable to grind the food. It requires quite a bit of skill to float teeth properly and recently it was in danger of becoming a lost art. Most veterinarians didn't want to bother with this as it's manual labor and seemed to them about on a level with being a blacksmith. Luckily, there were still a few old-timers who knew the technique, and they have now taught a new generation of "horse dentists" the method.

I tried to do everything myself around the barn, partly because I was interested in learning and partly to keep down expenses. One afternoon I was working on the off (right) hind hoof of a little mare that some smith, who didn't know his business, had rasped so that the frog (the horny mass in the middle of the sole of the foot) never touched the ground and the mare was virtually standing on tiptoe. As a result, she had developed a horrible case

27

of thrush under the overgrowth that had been allowed to develop. I was using Clorox to dry up the white, pussy discharge, but unless I could take off the heel of the hoof with a file so the mare could get a good footing, the Clorox wouldn't do much good.

The muscles of my brawny arms were more like rubber bands than iron ones and I wasn't having much success with the file when an old truck pulled in the paddock. An enormously fat man with blue eyes and thinning red hair had his belly hung over the wheel. Beside him was a spotted dog with a long tail who regarded me with cheerful interest. The fat man watched me critically, then removed the stub of a pipe he was smoking.

"Me name's Willy Bradley and Oi'm hearin' over at the Four Horsemen that you could be usin' a blacksmith."

I had said something about it to Mr. MacClay. With the mare's leg still in my lap, I threw back my hair and stared at him.

"Are you a good blacksmith?" I asked anxiously. After seeing what a bad one could do, I was worried.

"Better than that, I'm cheap." He got out of the truck and carefully lifted down the dog. Then to my surprise he walked toward me holding the end of the dog's tail up so his hind feet barely reached the ground. "Sam's gettin' a wee bit old, he was seventeen this May," he explained casually, "and his hindquarters are a plague to him." He let go of the tail and the dog instantly slumped down and lay still, but continued to watch everything around him. "Holy Mother, would ye be lookin' at that thrush! And who's butchered the poor baste's foot? Think shame of yeself, girl, and ask St. Francis, the patron of all dumb cratures, to forgive you."

I called on St. Francis and all the other saints in heaven to witness that I was innocent of the thrush. Apparently Willy believed me, for he took the file and went to work professionally. I sat and envied the swift, even strokes that corrected the position of the hoof.

Willy was good; even I could see that. After he'd finished the hoof and packed it with cotton soaked with Clorox, he gently pressed his fingers against the leg and stood motionless as though listening.

I knew people didn't like little girls jabbering at them when they were busy but I couldn't help asking, "What are you doing?"

"Sure, it's the pulse I'm takin'. It's a great thing entirely, the pulse. Fast or slow, strong or weak, thready or throbbin', when ye learn to read it, ye can be after tellin' at once where the trouble lies. Now Oi'll be takin' it in either hind leg. God gave bastes all parts in two's: two hind legs, two front ones, two ears, two eyes, and the like. So we'll check one leg against the other."

Willy showed me how to take the pulse. I have never seen it done before and, indeed, even today I have seldom seen a trained veterinarian who can do it. Although Willy was almost entirely uneducated, he had spent his life with horses and knew a tremendous amount about them. It was he who taught me to study a hoof for texture, water content, consistency, and color, and then to look at the shape. A horse may go lame from many causes and the trouble may be in the shoulder, knee, or ankle. Today, one of my specialties is operating on horses' feet to correct various conditions, and I have written a paper on the subject that has been well received; but I got my first training in hoof treatment from old Willy Bradley. I owe him a great deal.

After that, Willy was a regular visitor to our barn. I soon found that he lived in his truck; he not only had his forge there but also a bed and a crude kitchen. Like all smiths, he frequently injured himself handling red-hot irons or sticking nails into his hands while shoeing horses. Worried, I once asked him if he kept up his tetanus shots.

"Now what would Oi be doin' with the likes of that?" he demanded. "Devil a penny would Oi be spendin' for such. This is all Oi'm needin'," and he produced a pint bottle of iodine and poured it over a fresh cut. It made me wince to watch him. The iodine must have been a strong solution for it blistered his skin, but I never knew him to get an infection.

Having gotten a blacksmith, we were lucky enough to find a wonderful veterinarian. Dr. Allam was a tall, very slender man in his late thirties, always immaculately dressed. He carried his coveralls with him instead of wearing them everywhere as most veterinarians do. He would go to as much trouble over a little girl's pony as he would in treating a racehorse worth half a million. Mother just happened to pick his name out of the phone book and we were lucky. I'm afraid he was more amused than impressed by our efforts to operate a boarding stable, but he was such a kind man, he helped in every way he could. To me, a veterinarian was like one of the gods from Olympus come down to earth. I used to follow him about respectfully, watching in awe as he worked and never daring to ask questions. I noticed that he nearly always began by using a stethoscope and I often wondered what he heard that told him so much. One afternoon he came out considerably annoyed, saying, "Phyllis, I've looked everywhere for my stethoscope. Have you . . . ?" He stopped speechless, staring at a very red-faced little girl who had the stethoscope pressed against Flash's chest listening eagerly. Dr. Allam explained to me how it was used and then retrieved his instrument. That year my Christmas present from him was a beautiful new stethoscope.

Dr. Allam knew Willy Bradley well and said that he was an excellent smith and in great demand, yet I never saw Willy spend any money except for food for himself and Sam, his dog. I once mentioned this to Dr. Allam, who told me gently, "Willy's wife is mentally ill. Many years ago when they were both young, their only child died. She lost her mind and Willy has been keeping her in an expensive private institution."

I thought of Willy's old truck, his poor bed, and his life of hard work. I'd never realized until then how unfair life can be for some people.

Willy was always showing me some new trick in treating horses and in many ways I came to depend on him almost as much as on Dr. Allam. I had entered Flash in a show only to have him go lame the day before, as the result of a stone bruise. As it happened, Willy Bradley dropped in that afternoon and I sadly showed him Flash's bad leg. He examined it carefully.

"Now, that's no great matter. See, Oi'll be showin' ye a bit of a trick not everyone knows."

He got out his bottle of iodine, soaked a compress, and put it in the sole—the entire under surface of the pony's foot—and around the coronary band just at the top of the foot close to the hairline. "Keep it on for fourteen hours," he instructed me. "And when Oi'm sayin' fourteen, I'm not meanin' ten nor sixteen hours. Too small a time, and it's doin' no good; too long, and it'll blister. So have a care now."

The next day, Flash seemed completely cured. I couldn't believe it and was sure that somehow or another the judges would know he was lame and disqualify him. Much to my surprise, Willy turned up with Sam, as usual, riding beside him. For the first time, Willy was all dressed up and even had a diamond stickpin in his carefully folded cravat—well, anyway, it looked like a diamond.

"Flash is goin' to win a blue ribbon," Willy assured me. "And Sam and I are goin' to be there to see it."

We had fixed up one of Father's old trucks for a horse van, and with Father driving, we set off for the show. It wasn't a very big show; just the judging ring, a few booths, and a refreshment tent that sold beer and sandwiches. Still expecting the worst, I went into the ring with Flash while Father and Willy watched from the rail.

I had entered Flash in three classes: ponies over fences, hack, and musical chairs. I was so nervous that I made a fearful mess out of the first two. I got Flash off on the wrong lead, then realized what I'd done and made him break his stride, and was still worrying that his bad leg would show. I didn't get pinned in either class. Then it was time for musical chairs.

As I suppose everyone knows, in this class a line of chairs, one fewer than the number of contestants, is set up in the center of the ring and the riders ride around them while the music plays. Suddenly the music stops and everyone gallops for the chairs, jumps off, and sits down, except the unlucky person who can't find a seat. He or she is eliminated. Then another chair is removed, the music starts again, and so on, until there's only one chair left.

Musical chairs calls for good timing, rhythm, and perfect control of your horse, but Flash and I had worked together so long, I felt I had a good chance of winning. Round and round we went until there was only one other girl and myself. The music stopped and we both galloped for the remaining chair. I got there first and threw my weight back in the saddle to bring Flash to a dead stop, at the same time kicking my feet out of the irons so I could jump down quickly. Flash stopped so suddenly I wasn't

31

prepared. I shot over his head, turned a somersault, and landed on the chair. As the judge presented me with the cup, he said, "That was the most marvelous exhibition of horsemanship I've ever seen. How did you do it?" I replied modestly, "Well, of course, it took a lot of practice."

Willy was our smith for many years. A long time afterwards, after his wife had passed away, I stood by his bed in a nursing home and we talked about Sam and Flash and all the good times we'd had together. It was the last time I saw him, but I'll never forget how good he was to me and all he taught me about horses from his lifetime of experience.

That winter we lost Flash. He was very old and I'd known for some time he was growing steadily weaker. I'd seen plenty of sick horses; nearly every horse that came to my barn had something wrong with it. But I'd never seen death.

One evening when I went to his stall, Flash was down. I called Dr. Allam and he came at once, as he always did. "He's just too old, Phyllis," he told me. "But he had a good life and isn't suffering." Poor, dear Flash died an hour later with the tall, slender man kneeling on one side of him and a little girl in pigtails kneeling on the other, both crying.

"There's so much we don't know about horses," I wept. "It's not fair. They should get as good treatment as humans. When I grow up, I'm going to be a veterinarian and know all about them."

Dr. Allam didn't answer me for a while. In 1939 there wasn't a single woman equine veterinarian and the idea must have seemed ridiculous to him. At last he said gently, "Well, at any rate, dear, you already have your stethoscope."

2

FIFTEEN-YEAR-OLD PROFESSIONAL

By THE TIME I WAS FIFTEEN, I HAD PICKED UP ENOUGH KNOWL-edge about riding both from practicing with Flash and from listening to the men at the Four Horsemen to be able to compete in shows. I didn't have a horse myself but there were a number of people who couldn't afford a professional to show their horses, and so hired me. If it were a stake class—one in which there were money prizes—the owner would give me part of anything won. Otherwise, I was paid a flat fee. After I had partly gotten over my grief for Flash, I began to dream of getting another horse. But I didn't feel that it would be fair to expect Father to carry the cost.

My services weren't much in demand—then I had a lucky break. Ever since Willy Bradley had shown me something about horses' feet, I had been especially interested in hoofs and hoof malformations. These are a good deal more common than most people realize and at that time there was no known cure for them. Sometimes they didn't interfere with the horse's action, but in classes where conformation (the overall appearance of the horse) was important, any sort of foot deformity meant the animal was immediately disqualified. It was heartbreaking to see really lovely animals put down or discarded only because of this one fault.

That spring Mr. William Faunce asked me to show a mare

he'd just bought, one that had never been in the ring before. Mr. Faunce was a businessman rather than a horseman, although he kept two hunters and rode to hounds occasionally. Mother drove me to his estate, which was rather small but beautifully kept up, and his groom brought out the mare. When I saw her, I felt like crying from pure joy. She was the most beautiful, graceful creature I'd ever seen. Mr. Faunce was very proud of her, especially as he'd gotten her remarkably cheap, and the moment I began to examine her I knew why. Her left forefoot was deformed, like a human clubfoot. It didn't interfere with her movement but it ruined her looks.

"Can she jump?" I asked.

"I don't know. Why?" he answered, surprised.

"Because unless she can be entered as an open jumper where looks don't count, she'll never place," and I showed him the deformed hoof, which he hadn't noticed. No one should buy a horse without first having it vetted, but it's surprising how many intelligent people ignore this basic rule. In open jumping classes, only one thing matters: clearing the jumps. Conformation is unimportant.

I tried the mare out. She moved splendidly and you would never have guessed she had a deformity unless you looked. Still, judges have a nasty habit of looking. I tried her over jumps, but here the leg spoiled her stride and she would never make a jumper. For the show ring she was worthless—and I had to tell Mr. Faunce so.

He was greatly disappointed. "I'd like her to win just one ribbon," he told me. Later, he called in several experts, all of whom agreed that the mare would make a good, usable hack but wasn't show material.

I felt nearly as bad as Mr. Faunce. There was a show scheduled at the Stokes's estate in Berwyn, not too far from where we lived, which would have been perfect for her—not too big a show and not too small—if only it hadn't been for that poor foot. All the Stokes family rode and were quite knowledgeable about horses. They didn't maintain a big establishment but they had a beautiful show ring and everything they did was of the best.

The day before the show, we had one of those cloudbursts that I can't believe happens anywhere except on the Philadelphia

Main Line. The day had been hot and muggy without a whisper of a breeze. The leaves hung like dead men from the branches and the sheep and cattle stood under the trees, their muzzles almost touching the ground to discourage the flies. By evening, thunderheads appeared in the west, sharply etched against the dead blue sky. With them raced a wind that grew stronger every minute. As the storm came closer, the clouds were split by golden, zigzag cracks of lightning, almost instantly followed by the cannon crack of the thunder. The seemingly dead trees had become alive, swaying as if in agony as the wind tore at them and their leaves strained against the stalks trying to wrench free. A few drops of rain hit the windows of our house. The lightning was continuous and the thunder crashed down until it seemed to be coming through the roof. The raindrops increased and then came down in sheets. Cars had to stop, for the drivers could not see their own hoods. For perhaps half an hour it lasted. Then, when the storm had passed, the sun came out again, fresh-washed and brilliant, the air smelled clean and cool, and the birds began to sing.

The evening after a thunderstorm is a glorious period. Barefoot, I ran across our lawn where now there were a series of pools, some several inches deep. The gutters had turned into creeks and our lawn was covered with dead branches pruned by the savage wind. Sadly, I saw some grand old trees had been unable to stand against the storm and had fallen with their finger-like roots still reaching for the ground. Wherever there was no grass, the earth had turned to mud: mud so deep I sank into it over my ankles.

Suddenly, I had an idea.

I ran home and begged good, kind Mother to drive me to the Stokes's farm. The roads were running streams but we finally made it. I jumped out of the car and went to look at the show ring. It was just as I'd hoped: a quagmire. Not only that, all around it were pools of water and knee-high drenched grass.

That evening I called Mr. Faunce. "Please enter your mare in the Stokes's show," I begged. "In the hack class." The hack class is all on the flat; that is, there is no jumping. The horses walk, trot, and canter, and are judged on their performance. "And first have her shoes taken off. I want to ride her barefoot."

35

Mr. Faunce didn't ask questions. That was one of the nice things about him. He merely said, "Certainly, Phyllis."

Mother drove me over the next day. I'd taken special pains to be smartly turned out, knowing that that counts in these shows. My parents had had me outfitted by Brown & Co., which was then *the* tailor when it came to riding habits. I wore a blue-lined black jacket, white whipcord breeches, and a bowler hat. My shoes were Pearl boots, imported from London: very expensive but they never wore out. I had a cravat with a ruby stickpin. Father had explained when he purchased my outfit, "I'm going to get her the best so when she's in the ring, she won't have to worry about how she looks and can concentrate on her horse."

When we arrived, Mr. Faunce's groom was just unloading the mare from her van. I didn't want anyone to see her so I took her off by herself and rode through all the wet grass I could find— and I found plenty. Then I took her through several patches of thick, gooey mud, her unshod hoofs sinking deep into the mushy ground. When I'd finished, she looked as though she was wearing overshoes, the mud was so thick, and you couldn't see her feet at all.

Happily, I trotted over to the ring. There I had a terrible shock. Plunket Stuart's daughter, a girl a few years older than me, was there riding a truly handsome mare. And she knew how to ride. All the Stuarts did. Mr. Stuart was wild about fox hunting and early in the 1930s he had begun to buy up land in the Buck and Doe Run Valley, between Coatesville and Unionville. He wanted to keep it open for fox hunting. He brought over a pack of English foxhounds, which are much faster than our American foxhounds, and he and his family hunted three days a week. MFH Plunket Stuart founded the Cheshire hounds and fox hunt. This land is now bordered by the King Ranch from Texas and they run thousands of prime beef cattle there, fattening them up on the rich Pennsylvania grass before having them butchered, but it is still great fox-hunting country, perhaps the best in the East.

Miss Stuart was a famous rider and I'd often watched her at shows. She was, I think, the only person in the world I'd ever envied. Her mare was perfect and she handled her perfectly.

Well, I thought, there goes first place. I can't compete with that. However, I still hoped for a second or a third.

When the judge called, "Riders into the ring!" I was the politest little girl you ever saw. I hung back and let everyone else go first. I let them churn up the morass of a ring until it was over the horses' pasterns before I went in. The mare behaved beautifully and if it hadn't been for Miss Stuart and her lovely mount, I'd have felt sure we'd win. Finally we were told to line up.

I saw the judge coming forward with a bag. This was something new. As I expected, he headed for Miss Stuart. Oh well, maybe we'd get something. Then, wonder of wonders, he walked past her and handed me the bag. It was full of silver dollars!

I rode over to where Mr. Faunce was leaning on the rail and held out the bag. I was hoping he'd give me half, although often an owner gave a rider only 10 percent. Mr. Faunce, however, waved me away. "Keep it!" he said, smiling his pleasure. That bag bought a lot of hay and oats for my barn that winter.

That same afternoon, Mr. Faunce sold the mare to a man who had been impressed by her performance. Being strictly honorable, he told the buyer about her clubfoot, but the man wasn't interested in showing and only wanted a good, smooth-moving riding horse, which she was. Later, Mr. Faunce told a number of people about how I had managed to get his handicapped mare the blue ribbon—in fact, it became his favorite story—and I got a number of offers to show horses that had some fault or other. I was able to help several of them but I never again got a break like that miraculous cloudburst.

Because of this lucky chance, I became even more interested in deformities of the foot. I read everything I could find on the subject, though much of it was over my head. I made a nuisance of myself asking every veterinarian who would listen to me questions about horses' feet. And I was always told the same thing: that most often, nothing could be done. Yet I was sure there must be some answers, even though I hadn't the slightest idea what they were. I became more and more interested in horses' ailments. I studied every horse that came into our stable. I found bruised knees, spavin, bad hocks, ringbone, and some of the

37

animals were wind-broken. Dr. Allam showed me how to treat them all, and it made me proud to feel that I was doing some good. I also learned to recognize the early signs of foot deformity, and sometimes by special shoeing and rasping down of the hoof, Willy Bradley and Dr. Allam between them could allay the trouble, although it still couldn't be cured.

In my eagerness to help the horses, there were times when I did more harm than good. A woman had brought in a fine mare to be boarded and I saw the poor animal's legs were covered with ticks. I knew that kerosene killed ticks, so I bathed her legs in kerosene. It killed the ticks all right but the mare's legs swelled badly and her owner was naturally furious. She was fair enough to say, "I don't doubt your good intentions, Phyllis, but I do doubt your judgment." I hurriedly sent for Dr. Allam, who soothed the angry lady and assured her that no permanent damage had been done. He told me to rub the mare's legs with mineral oil and glycerin. In a few days she was all right again. But I'll never forget the scare it gave me.

Sometimes it was hard to know what to do, whether to trust my own judgment or obey the orders of adults. I had grown up believing that adults were right about everything, yet some of the people who brought in horses, although they were highly opinionated, didn't really know what they were doing. A few days after the kerosene episode, a man brought in a nervous gelding that had obviously been misused. The horse was so excitable it was several days before I could go into his stall. He was just becoming tractable when his owner returned and said he wanted to van the horse to some show. He asked me to help him and I agreed, although I knew that vanning that gelding was going to be a problem.

It was even worse than I'd anticipated. The gelding reared and refused to go up the tailgate into the dark interior of the van. If I'd known as much as I do now, I would have opened the front part of the van so he could see light ahead, but neither I nor his owner had that much sense. The owner was in the van, holding onto the halter and trying to drag the horse in by sheer strength, which, of course, was stupid as the horse was stronger than he was. Finally he said, "Stand behind him and hit him with a crop."

I didn't like this idea at all. I noticed this gelding had a habit of keeping his tail between his legs, which usually means a kicking horse. I got a crop and stood to one side. The gelding saw me and swerved away.

"That's no good," shouted the man angrily. "Stand right behind him."

I was about to refuse, then remembered how stupid I'd been about the kerosene. I stood behind the gelding and hit his rump. The next moment I was lying half-stunned on the ground, my face cut open and with a loose tooth. Even the owner was frightened. He thought I was dead. We never did get that horse vanned.

Adolescence is a hard time for a youngster. Sometimes you really do know more than adults; sometimes you get overconfident and make a fool of yourself. I was lucky in having a few adults I could always trust: my parents, Mr. MacClay, Dr. Allam, and Willy Bradley. For the rest, if I was told to do something I was sure was wrong, I'd try to temporize until I could get advice from one of my "trusties."

A short time later, I started my career as a "professional rider"—quite by accident.

The spring of 1941 Father had taken us all to the Garden State Track in New Jersey near Cherry Hill and just a few miles from Camden. This was amateur day, not one of the regular racing days. While we were there, a "powder puff race" was announced, meaning that only young girls could compete. Father wandered away, to return in a few minutes and ask me, "Would you like to race, Phyllis?"

I stared at him. I'd done some racing with Flash at shows but never at a racetrack. "I don't have a horse," I reminded him.

"I've been talking to a couple who'll let you ride theirs. She's a nice-looking little filly and I'll bet she's fast. Want to take a glance at her?"

Of course I did, although Mother looked worried. Already contestants for the race were beginning to line up, including several girls I knew. The couple was standing to one side with the mare tacked up. My impression was that they didn't know much about horses from the way they behaved and spoke. It's not uncommon to find people who like the idea of owning a horse

39

and attending shows but have no interest in horses as such; they just like the atmosphere of the track. The mare was a beauty, a chestnut a little over 15 hands. She seemed gentle and I was eager to mount. The couple was more concerned to make it clear that if I won, they'd get all the stakes. Father tried to argue with them but I didn't care. I just wanted to race.

It was a flat race, 5 furlongs and no gate. We all simply lined up and broke from a standing start when the starter dropped his flag. The little mare took off flying. For a few minutes, some of the other girls on bigger horses took the lead and I had to keep my head down to miss the clods that came flying back in my face. Then we pulled ahead. Not another horse came within three lengths of us from then on. After the race, the couple rushed over and while Father was helping me dismount, the man, in his excitement, turned around and kissed his wife. She stared at him for a moment, then said coolly, "That's the first time you've kissed me for months." I'll never forget her astonished look.

One of the girls I knew came over afterwards and asked, "Where did you ever get that mare? All you had to do was sit on her. You weren't riding her; you were just a passenger." I couldn't deny it. She was a fast thoroughbred. I've often wondered where that couple got her and what they paid for her.

Well, the couple collected the stakes as we'd agreed, and that was that. Anyone could have won with that mare. Still, I must have been doing something right, for afterwards I saw two men coming toward me. They didn't mean anything to me until Father whispered, "That's Danny Shea and his assistant, Fred Hammer."

I'd heard of Danny Shea all right. He was one of the most famous trainers in the East. He usually had a string of fifteen to twenty racehorses he was readying for the track for wealthy owners. I'd heard that he charged an average of $2,000 to train a horse and it took him anywhere from three to six months. Remember, this was in 1941, when the buying power of money was three times what it is today.

Danny wasn't an impressive-looking man like Mr. MacClay. He was a little Irishman, stocky, quick-moving, with a ruddy face. He seemed like a man in his thirties until you noticed the gray in his hair and the cat's cradle of fine wrinkles over his face.

His assistant, Fred Hammer, was a tall, slender man who wore a big, broad-brimmed sombrero rather like a cowboy's hat except that the brim was turned down.

Danny came over to us and introduced himself and Fred, speaking to my parents but looking at me. He complimented me on winning the race, and then asked, "Would you be wantin' a job exercisin' horses? I've never seen such a lot of ham-handed, thick-skulled, clumsy brutes as the exercise lads I'm cursed with. I wouldn't put most of them up on a mule, to say nothin' of a thoroughbred. Mouths cut, knees broken, tendons pulled. Yet I'm payin' top money for riders—seven dollars a day—and still can't get any who know their business."

I knew that exercising a racehorse is a delicate job. If the rider makes one mistake, he can injure the animal so he'll never make it to the track. With a horse worth tens of thousands of dollars, this is a serious affair.

I turned imploringly to my parents. Mother looked anxious, Father doubtful. To me it was a wonderful opportunity to ride top horses and learn about the track.

Fred Hammer said in the soft drawl of a Southerner, "How old are you, my dear?"

I gulped. "Fifteen."

"And what may your weight be?"

I hesitated a moment. I weighed 120 pounds but I knew that the lighter an exercise boy was, the better. "A hundred and fifteen pounds," I said with a straight face.

Danny nodded gravely. "You may not be havin' any experience but you know your first lesson. Always lie about your weight. Well, sir and madam, will you let us see how your daughter would do?"

"If Phyllis really wants to try it," said Mother, not too happily.

"How would you get back and forth between here and home?" Father asked.

My face fell. I hadn't thought of that.

"Oh, I'll drive her," said dear Mother, always ready to be helpful.

"Then let's see how you do. Jim!" Danny called. "Get Teddy Bear over here and put her up."

Jim was one of the exercise boys, a thickset, bowlegged lad

with big hands. Teddy Bear, to my indignation, turned out to be the lead pony. If a thoroughbred is too excitable or restless for a rider to handle, a line is snapped to his bridle and a man on the lead pony takes him around the track. Like all lead ponies, Teddy Bear was obviously a steady, gentle animal a baby could ride. I certainly couldn't exhibit my ability as a horsewoman on him. Still, I said nothing, and with Jim giving me a leg-up, I swung confidently into the saddle.

I heard Jim snicker and the men sigh. Danny said in disgust, "You come down on a racehorse like that, he'll take off like a goosed jackrabbit. The moment he feels your weight in the saddle, he's away. No, me lass, I'm afearin' we need someone who knows more about racehorses than you."

Fred Hammer said in his soft drawl, "Let me work with her a little, Danny. Now dismount and try again. Remember, get a leg up, go well above the horse, come down, and make first contact with your knees only. Then ease your weight down before you put your feet in the irons."

I tried again, although it was hard to get used to a racing saddle that seemed no bigger than a postage stamp. Fred was patient with me. I think his Southern background made him especially courteous to women. After several attempts, even Danny admitted that I might do, "if I can't get a good boy," he added hastily.

As spring was almost over, I didn't have to worry about school. We left home every morning at 6:00 A.M.—and I mean every morning, Sundays included, rain or shine, for the horses had to be exercised regularly. When we arrived at Garden State an hour later, I found my first horse tacked up, waiting for me. I had a string of six or eight horses to exercise daily around the mile-long track. After I'd mounted and was moving off, Danny would give me instructions such as, "When you get to the gap, jog first quarter. Gallop to seven-eighth pole, then ease off at a two-minute lick and break at the half-mile pole. Work him from there to the wire. I want him to go in forty-eight." The first time I got these instructions—which, incidentally, were to be followed to the letter or heaven help you—I wondered if Danny hadn't relapsed into his ancestral Celtic. It was Fred Hammer who saved me each time. The tall man with the funny hat would drift up beside me and explain softly, "When you reach the entrance to the track, go at an easy trot for the first quarter-mile. Then gallop him to the seven-eighth pole slowly with a strong hold. Then ease him out to a fast gallop. Let him pick up a little speed and at the half-mile pole let him go very fast. Keep him at this pace to the finish, but have him cover the distance in forty-eight seconds."

After a while I learned to distinguish between "breeze" (a fast but carefully controlled gallop) and "work" (letting him go all out). I also learned to judge time almost as accurately as a stopwatch.

There were good reasons behind all these detailed instructions. If a horse was galloped too quickly after he came out on the track, he wouldn't learn staying power; but if he was galloped too much, it would injure his wind. Until he was warmed up, he was uncertain on his feet and might fall. Each individual horse required a different treatment. Some enjoyed a gallop, others tried to run away and had to be held in by sheer strength; others again were lazy and had to be forced to step out. Some were "track sour" (disgusted with the whole business) and started stopping or slowing down as soon as they saw the track. You had to keep their heads up and force them forward. If they could get their heads down between their forelegs and arch their backs, you were in for a hard time. Others would run well alone but would refuse to pass another horse. I had one horse that developed the trick of lying down and refusing to move. This was dangerous as the horses following might ride over us. At first, I'd dismount and try to get her to her feet. Afterwards, I stayed on her and used my crop, forcing her to rise and lift my weight too. That cured her.

One of the worst tricks was "snatching the reins." The horse would get the bit between his teeth and abruptly jerk his head and neck forward. Unless you were ready for it, this could actually unseat a rider. You had to set your hands so that every time he tried this, he hurt his mouth, but immediately afterwards you had to relax the reins or the pain would make him rear or buck.

Some horses would shy. In my opinion, a horse should never be punished for shying unless it is obvious he is doing it simply to annoy you and perhaps unseat you. It must be remembered that a horse can see two images at once as he has eyes on either side of his head, very useful for an animal hunted by predators in the wild. A horse can, however, focus both eyes directly ahead of him, which in general is what a rider wants him to do in a race. A green horse first entering the race is looking everywhere but straight ahead. If you punish him for this, he becomes frightened, dreads the track, and is often ruined. If he shies at some unaccustomed object, you have to walk him up to it slowly and let him examine it. You must also remember that horses instinctively react quickly to anything unusual. In a wild state, they must do this in order to survive. Their senses are more acute than a human being's, and they can hear and smell better than we can, so a horse may be alarmed by something his rider knows nothing about. I also suspect, although I can't prove it, that to a certain extent a horse can read your mind. Of course, he can tell a great deal by your seat, by the way you hold the reins, and the pressure of your knees; but above and beyond that he often seems to know if you're confident, nervous, absentminded, or irritable. If you're afraid, your horse will be too. No one can absolutely tell what a horse will do. There's a French saying, "The only trustworthy horse is a dead horse." I don't like it particularly but I know what the French mean.

These thoroughbreds were big, powerful animals and my great problem was making sure that they didn't get away from me. Here the boys generally had an advantage, as they were stronger. I sensed this, and it worried me. Fred Hammer noticed my problem and he chose a curious way of correcting it.

There was a short-necked filly which I'd noticed the boys avoided and tried to keep from riding. It was soon apparent why. Our stable was nearly three-eighths of a mile from the track and sometime or other on the way to the gate, the filly would suddenly drop her head, spin around on her hind legs, and run back for the stable. Because of her short neck, it was almost impossible to stop her even when you knew of this trick. I'd studied this filly many times to see if there wasn't some way to prevent her stunt, but the boys put on her were the best riders, much stronger than I, and still they couldn't control the stubborn little animal.

One morning, to my astonishment, Fred called on me to take out this particular filly. I saw all the boys had big smiles on their faces. I knew that I couldn't handle the horse and I knew Fred knew it too, so I couldn't imagine why he wanted to see me in trouble. However, I didn't want to refuse so I got the horse tacked up and led her out.

Fred himself gave me a leg-up. As he did so, he said, "Wrap your reins around your hands and then cross them on her neck; lock them there. Then she won't be able to get enough purchase to spin. But remember, once the reins are on her neck, keep them there the whole time you're in the saddle. If you change your grip, she'll think it's a signal to start galloping."

Racing reins are heavy, rubber-covered leathers. I did as Fred told me. We were about halfway to the gap when the filly tried to spin around with me, but to do it, she had to get her head free. With the reins locked across her neck, she was pulling against her own mouth. Danny Shea was waiting for us at the gap. He looked at me a little curiously, gave me my instructions, and we were off. I followed orders and took her around in the correct time. The only problem was when I got back, it took me a couple of minutes to let go the crossed reins, I had them in such a grip. Fred held the mare until my fingers could relax. After that, I had more confidence in myself—thanks to Fred.

I had already begun to dream of being a veterinarian. I knew it would be an expensive business. It would take nine years—I'd found this out when I went to the University of Pennsylvania Veterinary School to ask about admissions. The woman at the admission desk said frostily, "Young lady, we have forty positions a year and we average 850 applicants. Even to be considered, you would have to have a college degree, which takes four years, and then a master's degree on top of that, making a total of five years' hard work, and with honors. So good day." I slunk away. I wasn't all that good a student and I knew my parents didn't have enough money for five years of college.

Still, on thinking it over, I decided to try. I worked harder at school and saved the money I was making at the track. I soon realized that there was no real future in exercising horses. I would have to become a trainer like Danny. Being a trainer paid well, plus the fact that a trainer had a chance to learn about horses while a rider or exercise boy only followed instructions blindly. Still, I had to be a thoroughly qualified rider and know all the tricks before I could hope to apply for a trainer's license. A trainer must be licensed by the state and must first pass two stiff examinations, one written and one oral, given by the Stewards of the Racing Commission. These stewards are nearly all former jockeys or professional riders and know every angle of the horse business. Even Danny stood in awe of them.

I had been losing confidence in myself because I wasn't as strong as the boys. When Fred Hammer taught me the trick with the crossed reins, I got back my confidence. That was fine except that soon I became too sure of my ability to ride any horse. I was overcompensating for being a girl in a man's world.

In addition to riding for Danny Shea, I also rode for other trainers at different tracks. One was at Monmouth Park Race Track, New Jersey. The man I rode for there was an owner-trainer, Colonel John Rutledge. He was very different from Danny. A big man with white hair and prominent blue eyes, he was gracious and charming, especially with people he wanted to impress. He had been a colonel in the United States Cavalry and was always irritated if you forgot and called him "Mister" rather than "Colonel." He was also a veterinarian, although he had lost his license. There was some mystery about him. He had come from Missouri with his wife a few years before and there were rumors that he had had to leave in a hurry, but why, no one knew. He had horses shipped in regularly from a dealer in the Middle West, and his wife, who was a splendid rider, showed them in the ring to prospective customers.

One of the colonel's horses was a big, strong gelding with perfect conformation, named Long John. He was brown, with a white blaze on his forehead and four white stockings. For some reason, he intrigued me so I looked up his record. He had never finished in the money, although he was always up with the leaders but in fourth or fifth place. I was curious as to what was wrong and asked Colonel Rutledge if I could try him out. He simply said, "Go ahead," so I tacked him up and went out on the track.

I thought that I could hold any horse with the crossed-reins trick, but Long John was something different. As usual, there were several other horses with their riders on the track and we joined them. I put Long John into a slow jog to get the kinks out of his legs. Then one of the other riders went past us at a breeze.

Long John became another animal when he saw a horse pass him. He broke into a gallop and then went all out. With the reins crossed, I tried to pull him in. I couldn't believe it. He might as well not have had a bit in his mouth. Whether at times like this he managed to get the bit between his teeth so it couldn't touch his lips, or whether he simply had a cast-iron mouth, I never knew. All I did know was that he was unstoppable.

By great good luck, I was on the outside of the track, furthest from the inside rail. Just as, by track conventions, horses are always ridden counterclockwise, so a horse being "worked" is always next to the inside rail. The next fastest is in the next lane, and so on to the outside, which is reserved for the worst horse— one that won't go straight or has some other fault. We were in this lane, but Long John was completely out of control. I finally had to admit it and shouted to the others to keep out of the way. When they saw it was Long John, they scattered like chickens. We went pounding around the track, Long John putting every ounce of his great muscles into his long stride. I'd never ridden like this and had no idea what would happen: he might fall and break a leg, or he might run entirely off the track, and where we'd end up then was anyone's guess. At a time like this, riders are more concerned about the horse than about themselves—I know I was—and I was trying to keep my head and think what to do. I kept my head fairly well, but I couldn't think of anything to do

There were two outriders watching the exercise boys around the track in case of trouble. One of them saw me. He was an old-timer who had spent his life at the track, as tough and hard as his stirrup leathers and nearly as thin. He put spurs to his horse, cut across in front of Long John, and picked me off the saddle just as they pick rodeo riders off a bucking horse when their time is up. By now, the exercise boys had reined in their horses and with no more competition, Long John gradually slowed down. When we came up with him, he was covered with foam and sweat, his mouth was open, and he was breathing in great gulping gasps. I walked him back off the track.

On the way, I met several of the exercise boys. One called to me, "Don't take it so hard. He's run away with all of us." Another said, "He's all yours if you want him, Phil. Nobody else will ride him."

At the gap, I saw Colonel Rutledge standing there watching. I said, "Why didn't you tell me he was a runaway?" The colonel shrugged and said, "He's potentially a great horse but if he's given a workout to get him ready for a race, he runs away with the rider and wears himself out. If he's not exercised, there's no way to get him in condition. I was interested to see if you could do anything with him."

I said, "Thanks a lot," and went on to the barn. I had lost a lot of my cocksureness that I could handle any horse, but I felt if I could master Long John it would certainly show I knew something about horses.

I thought it over for a couple of days, then took Long John out with a pony and stocksaddle for added security. I ponied him around the track for three days; by that time Long John had learned that he couldn't run away from the lunge line attached to his bit even if other horses were passing him. But no matter how much I ponied him, Long John was still a problem. If he ran away in the morning, you could forget about a race in the afternoon for he had exhausted himself. I didn't know what to do. Then the outrider who had rescued me that first day rode over to me when I was exercising Long John with the companion pony.

"I'll give you a tip," he said. "I've never told these boys about it because they'd break their fool necks trying it. You may break yours but you're lighter and have a better balance than they do. Shorten your stirrup leathers as much as they'll go so your knees are nearly up to your chin. When he tries to run away, stand straight up in your irons and pull the reins up. That will force the bit against his upper jaw and upper lip. Remember, you'll have to be standing clear of the saddle and pulling the reins directly up over his head. It's risky but it will stop him."

The first time I tried this, I thought I was going to fall off for sure. I couldn't grip with my knees and I had to balance myself as well as I could with a wild horse doing his best to run out from under me. I kept him as close to the rail as I could so he didn't have the whole track for his pranks. Then, slowly, I felt his head come up and I knew that I'd won.

A month later, the colonel entered Long John in an allowance race where the purse was $10,000. I should explain that there are two kinds of races generally recognized: an allowance race and a claiming race. In an allowance race, none of the horses is for sale. In a claiming race, any horse can be bought for a stipulated amount; that is, if the prize is $2,500, any trainer can put in a claim on any horse and buy him for $2,500. This is a curious arrangement but there's a reason behind it. Suppose you have a horse you want to race, but you know he's not good enough for one of the big races where there's a large purse that will attract some of the finest horses in the area. You put him in a race with a low purse, knowing that the best horses won't compete in such a small affair. But here's the problem. Someone with a fast horse may decide to pick up an easy $2,500 and enter his horse in the race under another name so the animal won't be recognized. In a claiming race, if he tries it, he'll win all right but he'll also lose his valuable racehorse for a mere $2,500. That keeps the race fair. After clocking Long John and seeing what he could do, the colonel decided not to bother with claiming races for small stakes but to try for the big money at once.

This decision made a lot of extra work for me and for poor Mother. Now we had to get to the track before dawn so Long John could be exercised when there was hardly any light. This was to avoid the "clockers." At every racetrack, there are men who sit there all morning with stopwatches in their hands, timing the horses so they can report their speed to bookies who lay the odds. As Long John had not been raced recently, the colonel could get very good odds on him if the clockers didn't know his real speed. Even so, by the time I was coming off the track, there'd be two or three men with their watches in their hands and one of them would call, "What horse is that, kid?"

I'd call back, "Captain, by Admiral out of That's Why."

We really did have a horse named Captain with those bloodlines who looked pretty much like Long John, especially in dim light. I'd ride back to the stables leaving the clockers industriously making notes.

Of course, Mother accompanied me every day to the track—I couldn't have gotten there without her—and her Pennsylvania Dutch conscience was bothered by this deceit. "Phyllis, you're not telling the truth," she reproved me one morning as we drove home.

Well, of course I wasn't, but it didn't bother me too much. I knew how much work Colonel Rutledge had put into Long John and how much money had been invested in him. The clockers hadn't put in any work or invested any money; they were just out to make a quick killing. My sympathies were with the colonel.

After a while the clockers realized that there was something special going on. Before dawn, they'd be fastened to the rail like crows around a cornfield. When the colonel saw that, he'd whisper to me before I started out, "Make it look as though you're working him for all he's worth but never get out of a breeze."

I always exercised Long John with three or four other horses. By now, we knew each other well enough so he realized that I could stop him if necessary, so he didn't try to pass everything on the track even if it killed him. I'd get behind a couple of the other horses and then make a great show of pretending to lay on with my crop and shouting, while making sure Long John didn't have his head. Colonel Rutledge would be there, watch in hand, with the clockers. When I came off the track, he'd shout, "Great going! That last was in fifty-two seconds. I'm entering him in a two-thousand-dollar claiming race next week."

School had started and this naturally cut into my time at the track. I was still able to exercise Long John and the other horses while keeping up my marks and no one seemed to object except my home economics teacher, Miss Kendall. Home economics was my only bad subject. I hated it. (To this day I have trouble sewing or cooking. If Mother and Norma weren't around to look after me, I'd live on coffee and sandwiches, although I might break down and learn sewing as I do like to look neat.) The woman who taught home economics was a great believer in discipline and also took for granted that every girl's ambition was to get married and be a devoted wife and mother.

I knew that if I ever hoped to be a veterinarian, I'd have to go to college as a preliminary to going on to veterinary school, and college meant a good record in high school. So I was as nice as I could be to the lady, even though there were times I felt like screaming at her to leave me alone. I think she felt that I was clumsy in home economics out of spite. I wasn't. It was like trying to teach someone who is tone deaf to play the piano.

One afternoon as I was leaving to exercise Long John, Miss Kendall stopped me. Even before she started talking, I knew there was trouble ahead.

"Your work in home economics has been most unsatisfactory," she told me. She was a thin woman with a voice that sounded like squeaky chalk. "I have decided to keep you in every afternoon until you have mastered a few basic domestic techniques."

I explained that I was expected on the track and that a good many friends and much investment depended on my getting Long John ready for the race.

She sniffed. "I can't imagine what interest you find in racetracks. There's no chance of your meeting a suitable man there. How you can expect to run a home and take care of a family with your attitude is beyond me."

I was late already for the track and I could see Mother outside in the car waiting for me. I lost my temper. "I'll hire someone to do housework for me," I snapped.

My teacher looked at me and her jaws snapped together.

"That, young lady, is an extremely impudent remark. You and I are going to see the principal."

I'd done it now. I couldn't afford a suspension or even a black mark on my record—it was hard enough to get into a college without something like that. I forgot my pride and was all ready to beg pardon, but one look at that narrow, hard face and I knew it would do no good. I followed her to the principal's office.

There was a bench outside where students sat waiting to be ushered into the presence. Except at assembly, we seldom saw the principal. To us, he was a combination of the Grand Inquisitor, President of the United States, and Lord High Executioner. There were usually two or three victims on the bench but this time we were lucky and went right in. The principal was a plump little man with tiny eyes surrounded by fat. He listened to what my teacher had to say and shook his head.

"Hanging around racetracks with grooms, stablemen, and gamblers? No life for a young girl! You were right, Miss Kendall, to bring this to my attention. It is disgraceful and lowers the reputation of the school. At Monmouth Track, you say? I know a little about the place—a haunt of the worst type of touts. And this girl is hand in glove with them, picking up their evil habits, learning their vicious secrets. Leave her to me."

Miss Kendall withdrew with a triumphant look at me. As soon as she was gone, the principal bent closer.

"Whom do you like for the fifth at Monmouth next Saturday?" he asked eagerly.

"Put your shirt on Long John in the allowance race," I told him.

Long John finished two lengths ahead of the field. I never had any more trouble with Miss Kendall and I still can't fry a decent egg.

3

GIRL MEETS HORSE

In a few months I would be old enough to get a driver's license, but in the meantime I was dependent on someone else to take me to the tracks. Most of the exercising had to be done early in the morning before the heat of the day, and this meant leaving the house at five o'clock to get to the track on time. Luckily, Norma had a driver's license, so all the burden wasn't thrown on poor Mother. We would get up at four-thirty, get breakfast, and Norma would drive to the track while I slept in the back of the car. It wasn't much fun for Norma but she never let me down. From six-thirty to ten-thirty, I exercised horses. I got $2 a horse. I was saving for college so the whole expense wouldn't fall on the family, but even with what I earned showing horses in stake classes, my bank account wasn't impressive.

Then I got a lucky break, or so it seemed at the time. I didn't realize it was almost to cost me my life. About 15 miles from Garden State Race Track where I was doing most of my exercising lived a retired dentist whose ambition in life was to own a racehorse. He had purchased eight unbroken colts more or less at random from various sources, hoping that one of them would turn out to be a racehorse. The colts were really wild: never been ridden or even halter-broken. He offered me $2 an hour to break them and get them ready for the track.

This was a wonderful chance to earn some more money toward my college tuition. I'd go to Garden State in the morning and then to the dentist's stable in the afternoon. Altogether, I rode about twenty horses a day. Of course, the unbroken colts were far harder to handle than the Garden State horses. While the dentist and his groom held a colt's head, I'd put on the saddle. At first, that was all I did, until the animals got accustomed to the feel of a saddle on their backs. Then I'd lean across the saddle until they accepted the extra weight. Next, while the colt was still in the stall, I'd mount, patting his neck and talking to him. When he came to accept me, I had the men lead him into the long, central aisle until I was finally able to take my nervous mount into the paddock. The whole process required about three weeks. Then I'd exercise the colts to get bottom on them—get them into condition—so they could compete in races.

The dentist had his own track, half a mile long. It was sand with a stretch of pine trees down the center, which meant you couldn't see across it. There was an outside rail but no inside rail. Still, except when it rained, it was a fair track. In a heavy rain, it flooded.

I didn't see much of the grooms but there was a stableman there who interested me. He was black and a giant, several inches over 7 feet. He had very thin features and never spoke— either he was dumb or he didn't know any English. He always wore a long raincoat that came down to his ankles. He avoided the other stablemen and grooms, who regarded him as a freak and made fun of him, although always from a respectful distance, for he was incredibly strong. I'd seen him pick up 200-pound sacks of feed and toss them around as though they were pillows. Even though he was clearly a loner, he and I seemed to have an understanding, perhaps because I was something of a freak too, a girl in an all-man's world.

One day there was a heavy rain, a regular cloudburst. It didn't affect the Garden State track especially but when Norma and I arrived at the dentist's barn, I saw his homemade track was a mess. Part of it had been washed away and there were several nasty-looking potholes. The biggest problem was that you couldn't tell exactly where the potholes were, as there were pools of water everywhere. The dentist and one of the grooms were ready for me as usual and had a colt already saddled. As I went over to inspect the track, I saw my black friend hard at work as usual; he was the hardest-working man I had ever seen. I waved to him and as usual he ignored me, although I always had the feeling that he appreciated my efforts at friendship.

After checking the track, I returned to the barn and told the dentist, "I'm not going to ride today. The track's too bad."

He was a little man with steel-rimmed glasses and a bald head. The horses had been doing well and he had clocked a couple who really did seem to have the makings of good racehorses, so he resented any break in their training. "Suit yourself, but remember, 'No ride, no pay,' " he told me.

I couldn't afford to lose the money so I told him I'd go ahead. The first two colts gave me no trouble. However, I noticed one place especially on the other side of the track concealed from the stables by the grove of pines, where there was a particularly deep sinkhole formed by the washout. It was a death trap for a horse, so I carefully avoided it.

My third colt was a chestnut, the fastest of all the string, but nervous and hard to handle. I jogged him at first and then as he seemed to be all right and steadying down, I let him gallop. He was going all out when we passed the hole. Suddenly a cock pheasant flushed from the pine strip and went roaring into the air beside us.

The chestnut was completely unprepared for the rocketing pheasant, which even to a person was alarming. By the worst of bad luck, he shied just as we were passing the pothole. He went into it. I tried to hold up his head but he went down. Usually when a horse falls with me I can kick my feet out of the irons and jump clear, but this time I went down too. I was pinned under him for a moment, then he was up and running, wild with terror. One of my feet was caught in the stirrup iron and I found myself being dragged along on my back.

This is the situation that every rider dreads. I had heard of several people who had died this way. On modern saddles, there is a release slip so the stirrup leather will come away in case such a disaster occurs. Unfortunately, this was an old, cheap saddle

55

and had no release. I could see his iron-shod feet lunging out toward my head and each time they struck, I was barely able to avoid them. I prayed for the leather to break but it held. I thought, *Dear God, I've nearly made enough money for my first year at college, I've worked hard for this chance, and now I'm going to be killed. It can't be true.* Only I knew it was true. I was weakening fast and in the next two or three strides the chestnut would cave my head in.

I twisted over and suddenly felt my foot come free. I lay on the ground while the colt galloped away. I was only partly conscious. I didn't want to move, I only wanted to lie on that warm, firm, safe sand. I was in a state of complete collapse, numb and helpless.

From where I lay, I could look down the track. I saw the tall black man slowly coming toward me. He looked as high as a tree. He stopped, gazed down, and then, surprisingly enough, smiled. It was a kindly smile as though he were trying to tell me that everything would now be all right. It was the only time I had ever seen any expression in his face. Then he picked me up as easily as I could have picked up a puppy and carried me back to the stables.

There was a crowd around the colt, anxiously checking him for possible injuries. One of the men glanced toward us and asked, "Are you all right?" I answered weakly, "Sure, I'm fine!" My black friend was the only person who had bothered to go looking for me or who was really concerned. He carried me to the car where Norma was waiting.

"Good heavens, Phyllis, what's happened? Are you badly hurt?" Norma cried, jumping out of the car. I was in such a state of shock I couldn't answer her. The stableman put me in the car, then left us. It was some time before I could tell Norma what had happened and that, except for the fright, I was all right.

The next time I went to the stable, I thanked my black savior. I don't know if he understood me. His face had resumed its usual expressionless mask and he turned away without making any sign. I spoke to several of the stablemen about him and they all assured me that he had never been known to speak or give any indication of understanding what was said to him. They took for granted that he was deaf and dumb. I never did find out the truth.

I was able to get a driver's license the following year and purchase a little second-hand Austin, so I could drive myself to the tracks and spare Mother and Norma. I now set about getting my trainer's license, which took a couple of years. I read everything I could find about horses and talked to everyone who would answer my questions. When I felt that I was ready, I had to find three trainers who'd sign a paper recommending me. Danny Shea, Colonel Rutledge, and one other trainer for whom I'd ridden signed the form. Then I had to apply on a certain day at the Racing Commission's office, Pimlico, Maryland. I was the only girl, all the other applicants were men. First came a written examination, then the oral. The steward and my examiner was a shrewd-looking little man, his face seamed with a tangle of fine lines from being used as a windshield for horses. He asked me a number of questions, several of them dealing with horses' ailments (here I think I knew more than he did). Then he asked, "Suppose you were told to get a horse ready for the track in thirty days. How would you go about it?"

I stared at him for a moment. "I wouldn't. There's no way to condition a horse in that short a time. They have to be built up gradually for at least three months."

The man made an impatient motion. "All right, but the owner is in a hurry and you're offered a big commission. Now what are the different steps you'd go about in the training?"

"I wouldn't take the job. It would ruin the horse and he'd be worthless."

"That's all you have to say?"

"That's all."

"OK, you're finished. Next applicant!" One of the men stepped up, and I walked away feeling miserable. Yet I still didn't know what I was supposed to have said. No trainer would undertake such a task, at least no conscientious trainer.

I'd obviously flunked and was getting ready to leave when my examiner, the racing steward, came up and handed me a paper. "You've passed," he said.

I stood speechless. "I still don't know how you'd get a horse ready for the track in thirty days."

"It can't be done. I just wanted to see what you'd say and if you'd hold your ground when I cross-questioned you."

So I became one of the three women trainers in the U.S.A. At nineteen, I believe I was the youngest.

Naturally, it wasn't too easy to find owners willing to entrust valuable racehorses to a green young girl, so I was delighted when an owner who was heir to a multimillion-dollar tobacco business and whose name is a household word asked me to get two horses ready for him. As this man could afford the best trainers in the business, I was greatly flattered. "I'll pay you ten dollars a day to train the horses and give you ten percent of the winnings," he explained. At that time, these were generous terms and I gladly accepted. This man was most kind and considerate, even drawing up a legal paper which we both signed to protect my interests.

Both horses were "brush jumpers," or steeplechasers; that is, they did especially well over wide jumps filled with brush. There was a particularly good brush course at the Laurel Race Course at Laurel, Maryland. With the owner's consent, I applied for two stalls in the stable there. There was no charge for the stalls (although there naturally was for the hay and straw), but if the association that ran the track didn't like you or your horses, they could refuse you stalls. Fortunately, there was no trouble, and I vanned the two steeplechasers to Laurel and got them settled down.

Laurel is a lovely little village and lives almost entirely on the track. Gradually, I got the horses in condition so they could be entered. In the first few races, both finished first and the owner scrupulously paid me my 10 percent. Then we started getting into bigger races where the competition was stiffer.

In addition to the brush course, there was an excellent infield track at Laurel where I used to exercise my two horses. There were usually several people using this track but as they were all experienced riders, this made no difference. One of the jumpers was a particularly powerful animal with a hard mouth, so difficult to stop, but he was a good-tempered fellow and we got along well.

I was exercising this horse one morning when there was only one other rider on the track. I had reached the three-quarter pole and let my horse go breezing along next to the rail. The horse and rider ahead of me were in the middle of the track so I wasn't concerned about them. Then, just as I reached them, the rider lost control of his horse, the animal turned sideways and began backing down into or toward the inside rail.

I knew that if two horses collided at that speed, something or somebody would be killed. I screamed and the horse ahead of me hesitated. We passed so close that his tail touched and slid off my boot! My horse was nearly as shaken by the experience as I was.

On our next race, this animal was still nervous and avoided the other horses, evidently expecting them to crash into him as the one on the track so nearly had. As a result, we came in third. There was still a sizable purse, and I went to the owner to collect my 10 percent. He told me, "Read your contract. It says get ten percent of the *winnings*, so you're paid if the horse wins." I checked and found that he was legally correct. I should have stipulated for 10 percent of the *earnings*. Here was a fabulously rich man who prided himself on tricking a nineteen-year-old girl. I don't know if that contract would have stood up in court, but I continued to race his horses for him, never getting my percentage unless we came in first. He finally moved away and I wasn't sorry to see him go.

I stayed on at Laurel. As I now had a little reputation as a trainer, several other owners hired me to train for them. I always rode the horses myself, never hiring exercise boys, so I would get to know the animals better. Every horse is an individual—some will work better in the morning than in the afternoon, for example—so each requires a different program. But in general, for the first two months, I saw to it that a horse was jogged for 2 miles and then galloped for 1 mile every day. It was not until the third month that I would let him be worked even for short distances. When working a horse, to test his ability I usually paired him with a known runner and then watched his style. Diet was important. I fed only the best Canadian Alberta oats and a mixture of timothy and legume hay. Most trainers use a great deal of additives, believing that they serve to "soup up" the horse and induce him to put out extra effort. I have used additives; there is nothing illegal about using them, but except in rare cases I never could see that they made any great difference. Usually they simply pass through the horse's system without having any effect.

I had not owned a horse of my own since Flash. Then one afternoon I noticed in Colonel Rutledge's stable a big bay gelding, 17 hands, ugly and ungainly yet giving the suggestion of great power. The colonel had connections with horse dealers from all parts of the country east of Mississippi, and although I had the feeling that some of these dealers were not the most reputable people in the business, they supplied him with an incredible variety of horses of all sizes, temperaments, abilities, and conformations.

The bay was crippled. He was broken down on his left hind ankle. The suspensory ligament seemed completely broken. Bad as it looked, the books I had read said that most horses recovered from such an injury if given time. For some reason, I liked the bay. His size, disposition, and intelligent eyes were all in his favor. I asked the colonel how much he wanted for the animal, knowing that every horse the colonel owned was for sale.

Colonel Rutledge smiled benevolently. "You have a true horseman's eye, my dear. A potentially valuable creature. Yet to you I'd let him go for five hundred."

"I only have three hundred," I admitted. He commiserated with me for losing such a great bargain. A few days later, he saw me looking at the gelding again and said suddenly, "Do you still want that bay?"

Like a little fool I said, "At the same price?"

I spoke too eagerly. As I realized later, Colonel Rutledge had decided to let me have the horse for $300, but seeing my eagerness, he changed his mind. He was really a friend of mine and wanted to do me a good turn. Still, he was first and last a horse trader. Without a change of expression he said, "Of course."

I agreed to pay $300 in cash and $200 in installments. The next day I vanned the gelding, whose name was Paper Cutter, to a stall at Laurel.

Dr. Allam had given up active practice and was teaching at the University of Pennsylvania Veterinary School. However, he was willing to look Paper Cutter over for me. "I believe he was once a valuable animal but he's been so abused I doubt if you can do anything with him. Why don't you see if he has any papers and send them to the Jockey Club? They'd tell you his background."

To my surprise, Paper Cutter did have papers. I sent them off and a few days later got an answer. My purchase was one of the great names in the history of brush jumping. He had won at Belmont Park; he had won a steeplechase race at Delaware Park; then something had gone wrong. He'd been passed from hand to hand until he'd ended in the colonel's stable.

With good care and rest, Paper Cutter's leg did heal. Finally, the great day came when I dared to try him out on the track. As his leg improved, Paper Cutter ran as I never knew a horse could run—for a while. Then he'd give up. Nothing could move him. I was convinced that he wasn't in pain. He was simply "track sour," that is, sick of the whole racing game.

I decided that Paper Cutter had been ill treated in races and so refused to take part in them, even to work out on a track. As he couldn't be exercised in the usual way, Norma and I walked him, every morning and evening, around and around the stables. The exercise boys thought two girls walking a discarded old horse's legs off was the funniest sight they'd ever seen. It took a long time, but at last Paper Cutter began to respond. He moved more easily and seemed to look forward to his walks. Yet we couldn't get him on the track and even on cross-country rides he went like an automaton. I tried every trick I knew without result. It was most discouraging.

Now that Dr. Allam had left, I had a new veterinarian named Dr. Bartholomew, a slender, white-haired, elderly gentleman with a lifetime's experience of handling horses. He examined Paper Cutter but could find nothing wrong. At last he said, "Get Paper Cutter to tell you what's bothering him."

I'm afraid that I didn't think this joke terribly amusing. The $300 that Paper Cutter cost had made a big hole in my tiny savings account and I was still paying Colonel Rutledge the remaining $200, so I wasn't in the mood for whimsy. Besides, it wasn't like Dr. Bartholomew to tease me or try to be funny at my expense. He was too gentle a person for that. I stood there solemnly trying to figure out what he meant.

61

The doctor finally took pity on me. "Stand in his stall door and watch him. He'll tell you what the trouble is by his posture, by his expression, by the way he moves and eats. You may have to watch him for some time before you'll finally find the answer."

Now I remembered that I had often seen Dr. Bartholomew watching a horse apparently aimlessly, sometimes for an hour or more. It had never occurred to me that there was any reason behind it; I had thought he was just idling away time.

I began watching Paper Cutter in his stall and in the pasture. What struck me especially was that he didn't appear to take an interest in anything. He ate without seeming to enjoy his food; he paid no attention to other horses or to people. Most horses when let out of their stalls whinny, shake their heads with pleasure, and go for a short canter or gallop at joy of being released. Paper Cutter never did. As far as I could tell, he couldn't have cared less where he was or what happened to him.

I could guess the answer. Paper Cutter had been regarded only as a machine to win races. When he failed to do that, he had been discarded. He had withdrawn into himself. He had only one real emotion: he hated racing. He had been pushed too hard, made to suffer too much spurring and too many whippings, until he had given up. Now he only wanted to be alone. Putting it a little differently, he didn't give a damn about anything.

I had to do something to wake up Paper Cutter and give him an interest in life. I'd been hearing a lot about hormone injections, which were just being introduced. I asked Dr. Bartholomew if they would help Paper Cutter and he burst out laughing. "Phyllis, dear, Paper Cutter is a gelding. Hormones don't work on geldings."

I went back to Laurel greatly disappointed, but having tried everything else, I still thought hormones might help. As Dr. Bartholomew was back in Philadelphia and anyhow considered the whole idea nonsense, I decided to get some hormones and experiment on my own. Unfortunately, to purchase hormones you had to be a licensed veterinarian. Still, there was a black market for such things around the racetracks. I'd never patronized the people who peddled drugs but now I took a chance. The $1.50 dosage cost me $20.

Amazingly enough, it worked. Within the next few days

Paper Cutter's eyes were bigger, more hazel, he had a better gloss on his coat, and his appetite improved. He still wouldn't breeze on the racetrack; racing had too many unpleasant memories. So I didn't push him. I let him set his own pace and run when he liked. As his confidence returned, he became more relaxed. Gradually he came to accept other horses when he found that he wasn't being forced to compete with them. In this, he was exactly the opposite of Long John, who was strongly competitive. Then I entered him in some minor races. Paper Cutter did well as long as he didn't realize he was in a race. When he thought he was merely having a pleasant afternoon run with some other horses, he was fine.

Paper Cutter wasn't especially fast on the flat, and I didn't really expect him to be. His record showed that he was a brush horse. Now, to my surprise and disappointment, he refused to jump, for no reason that I could see. I tried him at several stadium courses and he consistently refused. Then I remembered that he'd made his reputation "over brush." I decided to try him at that.

Cross country over brush is really a form of steeplechase and I think it's fair to say the most dangerous of all riding. The jumps are at least 4 feet high, often so high you can't see over them. They are also very wide. There may be anywhere between eighteen and twenty-one of them, scattered along a 2-mile course and deliberately located at the worst possible places: on top of steep hills, on the banks of a stream, around sharp corners. There is usually one "brush race" in the racing program daily at the major racetracks, as they are crowd-pleasers because they are so exciting. Horses are often hurt and sometimes lamed for life. The same is true of riders. As far as spills and thrills go, it's the closest thing to the ancient Roman chariot races.

Although Paper Cutter didn't like rigid jumps, he didn't mind brush in the slightest. He had a terrifically long stride so he could virtually step over most of the brush jumps, and when he couldn't, he simply plowed through them, being gifted with a cast-iron belly. I tried him in private over several courses and he came through nobly. Finally, I decided to enter him in a real race.

I was very crafty about it. I didn't dare enter him in any of the big, well-known races against really good jumpers, such as the ones at Delaware Park, ridden by highly paid, experienced professionals. I was too smart for that. But there was an obscure little race at Spring City, Pennsylvania, that I'd seen once or twice. It was an amateurish affair held in a cow pasture with homemade jumps, but the purse was $700. I could use that $700 with my college tuition coming up. None of the owners of good jumpers would bother with it, even if they'd heard of Spring City. So I entered Paper Cutter and myself in the cross-country "over brush."

Homemade or not, I knew the jumps would be tough and tricky and I needed the best tack both for myself and for Paper Cutter. I bought the best overgirth (an elastic girth that passes under the horse's body and over the saddle as a safety precaution in case the regular girth breaks) I could find, for the ordinary girth might not be able to take the strain of the constant jumps. It was so expensive that after I'd bought it, I was stone broke. I needed light boots. The galloping boots I used when exercising had long heels and were too heavy. Finally, I had to use my hunting boots. They were heavier than I liked but I couldn't afford anything else. On the morning of the great day, I loaded Paper Cutter into my homemade van and we drove to Spring City.

When I stepped out of the van, I had the awful sensation of having walked into a nightmare. All the top jumpers from the Delaware Park stables were there, ridden by professional jockeys. They had all reasoned as I did: it would be an easy way to pick up $700. Each owner, without saying anything to the others, had secretly instructed his grooms and jockey to take his best jumper to Spring City and enter him in the race. When they arrived and found all their acquaintances there too, they must have felt a little sick, but not nearly as sick as I did. Under the circumstances there was no chance of Paper Cutter's winning, but it was too late to turn back.

Paper Cutter had a couple of little peculiarities that made him an uncertain animal. Sometimes he still just quit for no reason at all. I didn't dare let him get away to a fast start because if he found himself ahead of the other horses, he'd stop dead and wait for them. I believe this was because he didn't like to feel that he was in a race. Also, horses are herd animals and in nature they normally stay together in a bunch, following the leader—usually the most powerful stallion—without trying to pass him. Some never get over this instinct. So I held Paper Cutter back at the start and we trailed the other horses the first time around the course. The course was bad, really bad, far worse than I'd fore- seen, and most of the horses didn't make it around. Paper Cutter with his fantastic stride and ability to stretch himself over wide jumps was now coming to the front, but if we were going to place in the money, he'd have to exert himself. I bent low on his neck and whispered, "Go boy!"

There was one way you could tell what Paper Cutter was going to do. If his eyes got big, he was willing to run. Now his eyes opened like the iris of a camera. I gave him his head.

He was so far behind that I thought he'd never catch up with the leaders, but several of them went down on the big, treacher- ous jumps that Paper Cutter took, quite literally, in his stride. He was an incredible brush jumper, possibly the greatest there has ever been, although he'd come down in the world to being ridden by a schoolgirl. At the last fence we caught up to the leader. This horse was a famous jumper and I'd never seen him beaten, al- though he was smaller than Paper Cutter, with proportionately shorter legs. His rider was a professional who knew how to get the best out of him. They were so far ahead that they must have been astonished when we appeared out of nowhere alongside of them just as they reached the last jump.

That jump was the worst of the course, high and very wide. With his long stride and ability to smash through brush, Paper Cutter always took off a little before he reached a jump to give himself plenty of space to rise to it. When the other horse saw him rise, he jumped too; but being smaller than Paper Cutter, he failed to make it. He came down two-thirds of the way across the jump, while Paper Cutter cleared it and went on to win.

Afterwards, one of the jockeys who'd been particularly sar- castic when Norma and I were walking Paper Cutter round and round the stables said angrily to a friend, "Sure that girl won. Anyone could have won with a horse like that!" He was right. Paper Cutter was a wonderful horse. The man just forgot that Paper Cutter had been discarded as worthless; he also forgot all the time and effort Norma and I had put into bringing him back. Later, I won both the Laurel and Pimlico distance races over brush with him, two of the biggest races in the East.

Mother, and to a lesser extent Father, were concerned that I was spending so much time at the racetracks. Garden State, Pimlico, Laurel, Monmouth, Delaware State—I knew them all. The racing world is really a world in itself, with its own language, customs, and people. Some of the people were rough but actually the only time you were in any real danger was when you were outside the track, not in it. All tracks were guarded by Pinkerton detectives, and everyone connected with the track had to carry identification and be fingerprinted. Once the gate had closed behind me, I felt perfectly safe.

In a world where huge sums were won or lost in minutes, there was bound to be a certain amount of crookedness. Not even the claiming races, which were supposed to be foolproof, were really so. An owner without much experience would buy a young, green horse and tell an exercise boy to see what the animal could do. Occasionally the boy would realize that he had an animal with great potential, but he would hold him in and then regretfully tell the owner, "I can't say much for that fellow. You'd better break his maiden for twenty-five hundred." This meant for his first race putting the horse in a claiming race with a small purse of $2,500. Often the owner accepted the rider's advice. Meanwhile, the rider would go to a trainer he knew and tell the man to put in a claim for the horse. Thus the trainer would get an animal potentially worth perhaps $100,000 for $2,500. Of course, the rider would be well paid for his trouble.

By now we had moved to an old Colonial farmhouse with a small barn in Berwyn, almost at the end of the Philadelphia Main Line. In those days—the early 1950s—this was real country. Although I was not a Catholic, my parents had decided to enter me at Immaculata College. Immaculata is first-rate, yet not as expensive as most, so I felt that I was very lucky to be accepted there. Mother was relieved that I was entering a religious university because she was still afraid that I'd be led into temptation at the racetracks. We both knew I needed the money but she would far rather have seen me earn it at the elegant shows on the

Main Line. The only trouble was, the purses weren't nearly as elegant as the people.

I had met a few Social Registerites at the shows. One of them was Henry Bartau. Henry belonged to one of the oldest, most aristocratic families in Philadelphia, and had a passion for animals of all sorts, even chickens and ducks. Far too much a gentleman to work, he was a gentleman jockey. It didn't pay much, but Henry was always able to find someone who'd let him live in a tackroom in exchange for keeping an eye on the stables. He'd make up a bed under the girths and reins and usually had two or three pet chickens that slept with him. In spite of everything, he was always impeccably dressed. Henry was invited everywhere and never turned down an invitation, especially if it meant free food. He was terribly good-hearted and looked after my barn in Berwyn when I was down at Laurel. When I offered him money, he was honestly hurt. He was glad to do me a favor, and besides, gentlemen in his position did not work for wages.

One of the biggest and most fashionable of the Main Line races was the Brandywine Point-to-Point. I knew that Henry was to be there as an outrider but I had no other interest in it, as it wasn't Paper Cutter's sort of race and no one had asked me to ride for him. Then, the night before the race, a woman I knew called and asked me to ride her husband's horse. As she was an excellent rider, I was surprised and asked her why she wasn't going to ride herself. She hesitated a little before saying, "I don't feel well."

I felt sorry that she had to miss the race and said that I'd gladly ride for her. I knew that Mother would be pleased that I was getting away from the bad influences of the racetrack and in among nicer people.

Norma and I drove to the hunt club. When we arrived, a man was just leading the horse I was to ride down the tailboard of a van. He was a big gray gelding and I liked the look of him, even though he seemed to be behaving strangely. Still, horses often do that before a race. I weighed in and needed a lot of lead to bring me up to weight with my little racing saddle. While I was tacking up the gelding, Henry rode over and studied my horse.

"Phyllis, I wouldn't ride that animal," he said quietly.

I looked at him puzzled. "Why not?"

"I don't like the look of him. Don't do it."

"I can't back out now. It's too late for the owner to get another rider."

At that moment, the owner himself came over. He had obviously seen Henry talking to me. Henry turned his horse's head and rode away, saying as he did so, "Remember what I say: don't ride him."

The owner was most affable and gave me a leg-up himself. In fact, he seemed reluctant to allow anyone else near the horse. As we moved off, he told me, "Keep his head up. Be sure you keep his head up and keep a tight rein. Stay behind the other horses—let them lead the way."

There was nothing extraordinary about these instructions. The horse moved well and easily. As we went toward the starting line, I saw the owner talking to a bookie. A huge pile of bills was exchanged. Clearly the owner was backing his entry to the limit; he must have great confidence in him. Yet suddenly I had the feeling something was wrong. I wanted to follow Henry's advice and dismount right there, except that the owner had been so pleasant I couldn't let him down. I was beginning to understand now why his wife had felt "sick."

The flag went down and we were off. My gray instantly ran away from the field. It was impossible to make him stay behind the other horses—he was going like a rocket. I'd never seen a horse run with a blind fury like this and it was a little frightening. We came to the first fence. As he went into his lead to jump, I had to relax the reins a little to let him have his head. He took the fence with a foot or more to spare: simply sailed over it. The moment he touched down on the far side, I tried to get him under control again.

I couldn't produce any impression on the brute. He had the bit between his teeth and was running away. I used every trick I knew, but it was like trying to stop a locomotive. It was uncanny. He didn't behave like a horse at all but like a machine. To take the next jump, we had to make a 90-degree turn—something most unusual in a point-to-point race. I pulled as hard as I could to turn him. The gray kept right on. In another few seconds he'd gone entirely off the course and was galloping all out down a dirt road, heading toward West Chester. I sawed at his mouth, jerked the bit, dragged back with the full weight of my body. Nothing I did had the slightest effect on him. For months now I had been training racehorses and plenty of them were big, tough, and determined, like Long John. This was completely different. The animal seemed to be mad.

Ahead I saw a four-lane turnpike with cars speeding along it, virtually bumper to bumper. My gray was headed straight for it. By a miracle of luck, an open field appeared on my left without fence or hedge between it and the road. I let go of the right rein and with both hands seized the left rein, pulling with everything I had, throwing all my weight into it. I felt the horse's head move slightly. I was desperate now, for the turnpike was coming closer. This crazy animal would not only kill himself and me, he'd also cause a major traffic accident. I jerked and strained on the rein and little by little his head came around. He left the road and charged across the field.

Even now he wouldn't stop. I was able to keep a strain on the bit so he went in circles. He was foaming at the mouth—great gobs of saliva as thick as froth from a dishwasher. It kept flying off and hitting me in the face until I was blinded. I knew enough to realize what that meant: he had been drugged. This explained his mad behavior. He *was* mad.

The saliva was coming out of him in what seemed to be bucketfuls and I was so plastered with the stuff that I could no longer see where I was going. I must have relaxed my grip on the reins, for he straightened out and went at full gallop into a tree. The shock threw me off his back and I landed on my feet, grabbing the reins. He was standing still now, his head sunk between his forelegs. Somehow I got him turned around and led him back toward the hunt club.

It was a 2-mile walk, but long before we got there I met Henry Bartau, who had come to look for me—or what was left of me. It was a tribute to his concern that his first question was, "Are you all right?" rather than, "Is the horse all right?" Usually people ask after the horse first.

I said, "Yes, I'm fine," which was a terrible lie.

"How did you stop him?"

"Easy. I ran him into a tree. I think he has a concussion. Better get him to a vet fast."

"And you'd better get to a doctor."

Henry took the horse, who was now staggering and quite subdued, while I went on alone. I was shaking and felt weak around the knees. Norma was waiting for me at the car. She took one look at me and asked, "What happened?"

I told her as I fell into the car. "Do you think I should apologize to the owner for not finishing the race?" I asked weakly.

Norma snapped, "I think you should have him put in jail, but don't worry about that now. I'm getting you home." When we reached home, I went to bed.

I am convinced the drugged animal would have won easily except for that unexpected 90-degree turn. Unlike the racetracks where there's pari-mutuel betting and the horses are carefully checked for doping, these society events were not supervised, it being taken for granted that elegant ladies and gentlemen would not stoop to such methods. Well, enough of them stooped so that today all horses are checked when there's a substantial purse offered.

When Mother got home that evening and spoke to Norma, she hurried upstairs to see me. I said weakly, "From now on, I think I'd be safer with all those rough characters at the tracks." Mother made no reply except to ask how I was. From then on, I never accepted a mount again until I'd tried him out and made sure he wasn't drugged.

4

STATE CHAMPIONSHIP

BEFORE I COULD ENTER VETERINARY SCHOOL—IF I EVER DID—I
would first have to graduate from college with several credits in
biology and be able to read and write at least one foreign language; this, of course, in addition to my other college credits. I
was glad to be going to Immaculata College, both because of its
high scholastic reputation and because I could live at home and
commute, thus saving me the considerable cost of boarding.

Unfortunately, Immaculata had no course in comparative
anatomy, which I needed in order to enter veterinary college. I
was saved by one of the nuns who taught physics and chemistry.
She didn't know any more about comparative anatomy than I
did, but she got a book on the subject and studied it. I was her
only pupil in the course and I think she stayed one day ahead of
me, reading the next day's lesson every evening. It was necessary
for me to dissect the dead bodies of cats that had been injected in
a certain way so the veins were a different color from the muscles. This kind woman provided the bodies, using, as I later
found, her own money, as there was no budget in the college's
resources for such equipment. For my language, I selected German but would probably have flunked if it hadn't been for a
Dutch girl who was attending the college. This girl spoke fluent
German and spent long hours tutoring me. She was always jolly
and lighthearted until one day she broke down and told me how,

71

after the Germans had invaded Holland, they had come to her village and taken away all the men and most of the women. She and a few others had escaped. Those whom the Germans had taken were never heard from again. She wept as she told me the story and for the first time I realized what an easy life I had. That girl and the kind-hearted nun nursed me through Immaculata.

In spite of my troubles and the discouraging attitude of the woman in admissions at the veterinary school, I never doubted that some day I would be a veterinarian. There was a tower at Immaculata where I used to go when I wanted to be alone. There I could sit in the window niche looking out over the Great Valley —that huge, fertile rift running from Lancaster to the suburbs of Philadelphia. The Indians used to call it the "Dark Valley" because it was so thickly overgrown with trees and brush; now it is mostly farmland. From the tower I could see Swedesford Road, once the Minquas Trail made by the local Indian tribe, and Conestoga Road, where the original Conestoga wagons took the pioneers westward. On the far side of the valley ran Bacton Hill, a long ridge with the oldest landmark recorded in the area, Little Rough Top, where the sandstone thrusts up through the limestone covering. It is shown on the earliest survey map made in 1681. Almost directly below me was Warren Inn, where the British plotted the Paoli Massacre, and a few miles to the west the old General Wayne Inn, where you can still see the marks of the teamsters' whips on the back of the door when they tried to snap off nails with one crack. At the corner of Bacton Hill Road and Swedesford Road there was still a blacksmith's forge in operation, just as it had been ever since the Revolution, and near it the White Horse Inn, now a private house. I'd sit there and dream of the time when I would be a licensed veterinarian driving my car from farm to farm, stable to stable, show to show.

I think my parents believed that my interest in horses would pass or at least I'd be content with being a rider or a trainer. But I wanted to do something really important with horses if I could. I'd noticed that often young maiden mares are infertile, no one knew why. Also I'd seen a number of older brood mares with irreplaceable bloodlines that had stopped conceiving. The veterinarians usually told their clients, "Too old. Put her down and get a young mare." I believed that most of them could have had another couple of foals if we knew more about how reproduction in horses worked. We were just beginning to learn something about hormones. It was a whole new field.

When I first told my family that I intended to become a veterinarian, Mother was the enthusiastic one. I could have announced that I was planning to fly to the moon and she would have started laying the launching pad in the backyard. Father shook his head, looked doubtful, and then as usual was his practical self. "Well, let's see how you can go about doing it," he said.

I knew it would be hard going, but I didn't realize how hard. In the early fifties there was considerable prejudice against women going into what was considered "men's fields." I became especially conscious of this feeling when, after I'd gotten my master's degree at Immaculata, I went to the dean of the University of Pennsylvania Veterinary School to submit my application for admittance. The dean was Dr. Kelser, a man in his sixties with a big, florid face and an abrupt manner. He was a former Army veterinarian and a great believer in discipline, and he had a rather low opinion of women. He scowled at me and bellowed, "What would a hundred-pound girl like you do if you had to handle a thousand-pound bull?" I retorted, "Exactly what a two-hundred-pound man like you would do—I'd sedate him." For a moment, I thought Dean Kelser was going to jump up, grab me by the nape of my neck and the back of my skirt, and throw me out. Instead, he stared at me for a few seconds, then said, "Your application is accepted." I afterwards found that Dean Kelser might be tough but he respected anyone who stood up to him.

Yet a few weeks later, I nearly gave up all idea of ever becoming a veterinarian. Dr. Bartholomew had once called me pigheaded and plenty of people agreed with him, but the more I thought about veterinary school, the worse the odds looked. Even the people who knew and liked me—like Dr. Bartholomew and Dr. Allam—seemed to think that no woman could make the grade as an equine veterinarian, which was my ambition. Dogs and cats, yes, but horses were too big and powerful for a woman to handle. I was a good student though not a brilliant one, and to qualify I would be in the competition with some of the best

73

students in the eastern United States. Worst of all was something Dr. Bartholomew had said. He had warned me, "Phyllis, you're crazy over animals, especially horses, but as a veterinarian, you'll have to cease to be an 'animal lover' and become a scientist. You're spending far too much time with horses now."

"If I'm to be an equine practitioner, how can I spend too much time with horses?" I protested.

"Horsey people aren't scientists; they don't have the temperament for it. Scientists think and live in a different world from the horsey people. You're going to be a scientist. You must think of a horse as though it were a machine that has broken down and needs fixing."

But I couldn't think of horses as machines and I didn't want to try. I loved riding. It was my life.

At this crucial moment, a wealthy woman who had a magnificent stable came to me with a proposition. She had seen me ride in a number of shows and I had exhibited some of her horses for her with good results. She wanted to take me on as a full-time trainer, working only with her string. The salary would be $500 a week. In terms of today's buying power, you can multiply that by three. She also offered me a cast-iron contract for the next five years. I was twenty-one.

With all my doubts and fears about veterinary school, this was too much. I told my parents that I'd decided to accept the job.

I couldn't believe it when they both urged me not to do so. I'd taken for granted that they'd be delighted if I took this high-paying job. "No matter how much you're paid, you'd be that woman's servant, with no future," Mother pointed out. And Father added, "You've always wanted to be a veterinarian. There you can really amount to something and perhaps make a real contribution to medical knowledge."

I thanked the lady and told her I couldn't accept her generous offer. A few weeks later, in some way that is a mystery to me, she went bankrupt, lost her stables, and vanished. I never knew what became of her.

Although Dean Kelser had accepted my application, it still had to be approved by a committee. Through some veterinary friends I knew who were connected with the school, I learned that only one member of the committee wanted to see me admitted: Kelser himself. I met the dean occasionally and I got the impression he was growing increasingly discouraged. At last he told me, "If you don't hear by April, you've been turned down."

I went on with my usual tasks, rushing out to meet the postman every morning. April came and was nearly over. Still no word.

One morning listening to the radio while mucking out stalls I heard the program interrupted for a special announcement. "I regret to inform you," said the commentator, "that Dean Kelser of the University of Pennsylvania Veterinary School died this morning of a heart attack."

It was one of the greatest shocks of my life. I felt Dean Kelser's loss deeply. In spite of his gruff manner, he had been good to me and I knew he had gone out of his way to help me—almost surely against strong opposition. It was also a ruinous blow to my hopes. Without his support, I had no chance at all of getting into veterinary school. Five years and thousands of dollars wasted.

I finished the stalls, working automatically, then from force of habit went to the mailbox. There was one letter in it, from the college. Still in a state of shock, I took it out and opened it. It was my application, approved by the committee and signed by Dean Kelser. It must have been almost his last act.

From here on, everything seemed smooth. It was the end of summer. The day was Friday and veterinary school opened on Monday. We were boarding a mare, a fine racehorse who had been fired a few days before. This process sounds cruel and it is now going out of fashion, although it is a very ancient technique. A hot iron is used to build up scar tissue and toughen the ankle. I still think it is the only treatment for certain conditions. The mare kept pulling at her sore ankle, so a cradle—a sort of collar made of many wooden slats—had been put on her neck to prevent her from reaching her leg. I noticed that the cradle had slipped and went in to adjust it.

Suddenly the mare threw up her head and the cradle struck me full in the face. I was flung against the side of the stall and fainted. When I came to, I was lying on a pile of bloody straw, hardly able to see and too weak to stand. I crawled out of the stall on my hands and knees and lay semi-conscious in the aisle until Father found me. He rushed me to a doctor who sewed my head up, but I was still dizzy and had trouble seeing clearly.

I was able to report to veterinary school on Monday but I could hardly read print, let alone see through a microscope, and our first lesson was an introduction to microscopic work. My headaches got increasingly worse, and most terrifying of all, my eyes were failing rapidly. At last, there was no choice; I had to go to the new dean and asked for a year's medical leave of absence. He told me, "I'm sorry, but if you leave now, you won't be reinstated." So I stuck on.

By January, I could take it no longer. I was falling behind in my studies and could not see well enough to read a book. I had to drop out. When my doctor examined me, he said, "Don't worry about veterinary school. You will take a long, long time to recover."

A few days later, I heard Father and Mother talking together. The doctor had spoken to them and said that there was a strong possibility I would be permanently blind.

The next few weeks were the worst in my life. For the first time I lost hope. My family was heartbroken and didn't dare discuss my blindness with me. I wasn't permitted to use my eyes at all, not even to skim through a book or look at a newspaper. In one stupid moment of carelessness I had destroyed my life and thrown away the time and money my parents had sacrificed for me. The special preparatory school, college, and all my efforts to enter veterinarian school had been wasted.

To me, the threat of blindness was the most terrible of all fates. After all my great dreams and ambitions I could well end as a burden to my family, unable to do anything but the simplest tasks. If only I had been a little more careful when I adjusted that rigid neck cradle. It was entirely my own fault; I had no one to blame but myself. Dr. Bartholomew, Colonel Rutledge, Henry Bartau, and even Danny Shea and Fred Hammer had warned me repeatedly to be more careful when I worked with nervous, high-strung animals, but I had always managed to quiet even the most aggressive, and had grown overconfident. I told myself that if I ever recovered my sight, I would never take chances again.

Slowly my vision returned. Three months after my accident, I could read large print. Then I was able to read a newspaper. I still didn't dare use a microscope, but I was getting better.

It was nearly a year before my sight returned to normal and I was able to save up enough money for my tuition and extras. I have always hated to ask for favors and have perhaps been a little too defiant about my independence, but this time I was desperate. I wrote the most humble letter of my life to the dean of the veterinary school. I knew my instructors had felt that I was spending too much of my time at the racetrack and working with horses rather than with my books. In my letter, I said that if I could only return to the school, I'd never go near a horse until after I had graduated. I'd give up riding and keep away from horse shows. For answer came a letter reinstating me and also assigning me a room in the dormitory. The dean added a note: "I think it would be a good idea for you to live on campus so you won't be tempted to sneak away to the stables and get involved with dangerous horses again." I accepted his terms gratefully.

In the dormitory I had a roommate, a girl my own age named Elaine Hopkins who was also studying to be a veterinarian. She intended to work with small animals. We were getting into the age of specialization, which has now been carried so far that often a veterinarian who works with dogs won't treat cats, and vice versa. This isn't as crazy as it sounds as cats react strongly to certain drugs that are quite suitable for dogs and other animals. It is difficult to anesthetize a cat; they die easily and both morphine and occasionally ether have a violent effect on them. I myself would never treat one; it's too much of a restricted field.

Elaine and I became great friends and have remained so, even though we are unlike both physically and mentally. She was brilliant, with a high I.Q., a big girl, and when nervous, as just before exams, tended to eat enormously. I am very average academically, slender, and when I'm nervous, I can't eat at all. I have to force myself even to drink coffee. Elaine was full of fun and could see something funny in nearly everything, while I'm more serious. I was devoted to just about the biggest of domestic animals, horses, while the hearty Elaine loved the smallest: dogs and tiny, caged birds. Her hands were wonderfully deft and she had a collection of almost microscopic surgical instruments for operating on canaries and finches, which she did with amazing skill.

It was through Elaine that I got my first patient. Both of us were hard up, as were most of the students, and one day Elaine marched into our room with the good news that she had an operation lined up for us that paid all of $15. I was delighted, but reminded her that we weren't licensed veterinarians.

"Oh, it's a very simple operation—just deodorizing someone's pet skunk," Elaine answered lightly. "My father showed me how to do it once. The trick is to pick the skunk up by the tail, then he can't squirt you. You just have to be quick, that's all. I thought I'd let you do that part."

"You're all heart," I assured her. Still, fifteen bucks represented seven hours of riding half-broken colts, and how bad can a skunk smell anyhow? I was to find out.

The skunk's owner lived a few blocks from the veterinary school and we went down in Elaine's car with our equipment. The owner turned out to be a fat man with flashing glasses who was obviously known as the life of the party. "Stinker always creates a sensation when he walks into a room," he assured us, as he led the way toward the kitchen. "All he has to do is stamp his forefeet and raise his tail and people go straight out the window."

Stinker was about the size of a large cat, with rich, glossy, ebony fur, a double white strip running down his back, and a magnificent tail over one-third of his entire length. Although a little too low-slung to be considered graceful, he marched up to us in an impressive, flat-footed manner, obviously sure that everyone would get out of his way.

"I'll leave you two alone with Stinker for the operation," said the man. "Be gentle with him," and he left us.

"All you have to do is to be quicker than Stinker," said Elaine briskly. "One quick grab and you have him."

I approached Stinker cautiously. Before setting out on this project, I'd done a little reading on skunks. A skunk's musk is not simply a bad-smelling substance; it is a powerful acid known technically as mercaptan. It has an ammonia base and can produce permanent blindness. There is one case on record of a man who got a full dose of musk in the face at close range and died from the effect. Even when the musk lands on your bare skin, it can produce painful burns. The reason a skunk is so plainly marked in black and white is so other animals can immediately recognize him and keep clear; otherwise he'd be constantly wasting his precious musk as skunks are slow-moving and perfectly fearless.

I knew from my research that the musk is discharged from two ducts that the skunk protrudes from the anus to make sure he doesn't get any of it on himself. So I reasoned that as long as I kept in front of Stinker, I was safe. I took another step. Up went the tail. With the tail out of the way, Stinker was obviously ready to shoot from the hip, but he still faced me. I reached down. The white tip of the tail fanned out. I made a grab for it.

Stinker looked clumsy, but with amazing quickness he twisted himself into a U and fired just as I got his tail. Luckily, he didn't hit me in the face. The musk struck my white coveralls a little above the belt. Musk has been described as a combination of ammonia, garlic, sulphur, sewer gas, and vitriol, all raised to the nth degree, but words fail to do it justice. Both Elaine and I gasped for breath, our eyes burned and ran, and I felt sick at my stomach.

"Put him on the table," said Elaine hoarsely, for the musk affects the vocal chords. I got Stinker back of the neck as he was trying to bite me and laid him on the table. A skunk can fire several times before he runs out of musk and Stinker did. I don't know how his owner ever deodorized the kitchen but that was his problem.

With a young skunk, removing the glands is a comparatively simple matter—but Stinker was full-grown. It takes some skill to differentiate between the glandular and muscular tissue, and if the rectal wall is cut, it will not heal. Elaine worked swiftly and well.

We got our $15. As we were leaving, Elaine asked the man in her new, hoarse voice, "How do you clean a suit of clothes that has been skunked?"

"There's only one sure way," the man told her. "Soak them in tomato juice, wash them with lye and carbolic soap, and then bury them—and leave them buried. Ha-ha-ha!"

We found out he was right. Deodorizing Stinker cost us both a suit of coveralls because Stinker had managed to nail Elaine while he was stretched out on the table. No matter what we tried, our coveralls still smelled. That was the last time I ever deodorized a skunk. I decided to stick to horses.

During my last two summers in veterinary school, I was required to intern with a recognized veterinarian. My dear old Dr. Bartholomew had long since retired, so I had to look around for someone else—someone who would take me and whom I liked. I finally decided on a racetrack veterinarian named Dr. Charles. Dr. Charles was an excellent veterinarian who knew a great deal about horses and inspired confidence, but that was only part of the reason I was eager to work under him. I was shy and did not get along well with people. I had learned that being a good doctor is only part of being a successful veterinarian. You had to make friends and get people to trust you. Dr. Charles was expert at both. He was a little man, only 5 feet 6, and always dressed impeccably in a gray charcoal suit, shoes shined to a high gloss, his neat mustache carefully trimmed. He hardly ever wore the coveralls that were virtually a uniform with most veterinarians. He was a good talker, always jolly and friendly, and spent a great deal of his time in bars at the various tracks, not doing much drinking but always talking and buying owners drinks. He was enormously successful and I felt I could learn a lot from Dr. Charles.

I was too shy to ask him if he would act as my sponsor, so Father did it for me. I did not realize it at the time, but Dr. Charles would have refused had he dared. I don't think he disliked me; he simply did not want to be bothered. But he owed Father a great many favors and wanted still more from him, so he said that he'd take me. I was delighted.

Dr. Charles was my first experience with a veterinarian who was primarily a businessman rather than a doctor. I don't believe that he had any true medical interest in horses whatsoever. His practice at the racetracks was limited but highly remunerative. The ailments were always the same, so a veterinarian's duties were repetitious: lameness problems, wind examinations, blood tests, vitamin injections, over and over. We were usually finished by noon, then spent the rest of the day socializing with the owners and trainers, a vitally important part of his practice. I found it terribly boring, especially as I was interested in widening my experience in other medical areas, fields that did not pay as well as the routine doctoring of valuable thoroughbreds. Dr. Charles ignored them.

I recall one incident that hurt me deeply. One of the horses I was boarding had a slight nasal discharge and I asked Dr. Charles if he would look at the animal. He was in his car with his assistant, a man with no medical knowledge whatsoever. He turned to his helper and said, "Give the kid's horse a shot of penicillin. That's probably all it needs." He did not even bother to get out of the car himself to look at the animal. When his helper returned, he said to me, "That will be twenty-five dollars. I don't work for nothing, you know." I marched into the house and got him the money, which he pocketed without comment. I never asked his help again.

I had approached veterinary medicine with an idealistic attitude. Being under Dr. Charles was a valuable experience as it showed me how a hard-headed, highly practical man operated. I thought he had no interest in me and neither knew or cared how I felt, but when the time came for us to part, he gave me an excellent piece of advice, which showed that he knew me better than I realized. He said, "Phyllis, I'd keep away from the racetracks if I were you. You've got a good family, a good education, and friends. Take advantage of them. I never had a home or a family. I was always on my own. Being a racetrack veterinarian and living out of a suitcase, eating in restaurants, and spending your life in bars is too hard a life."

I followed his advice. Being a racetrack practitioner is indeed too limited; also you see too many heartbreaks. A man may come to the track with one or two horses on which he's spent all his savings and in a week or a month he's lost everything, even the horses. Racing is too impersonal for me. I never enjoy watching it unless I know one of the horses personally and want to see how he'll do.

It is strange how often some seemingly casual chance event changes the whole course of your life. This has happened several times to me. Perhaps it happens to everyone, I don't know. That summer turned out to be one of the most important in my life.

A man who was boarding a horse at my stable asked me to go down with him to Dover, Delaware, to look at a mare and see how I liked her. It was late in the afternoon, I was so tired that I could hardly drag myself around, and the last thing I wanted to do was drive all the way to Dover and back. Still, I didn't want to be rude, so I said that I'd go.

The stables were not impressive and neither was the mare. She was a little brown animal standing 15 hands 2 inches. It was hard to know how to place her. I was sure that she was too small to be a good open jumper, which was what my friend wanted; on the other hand, her conformation was not good enough for a show hunter. As long as an open jumper can jump anything that comes along, she can look like a camel and it makes no difference; but a show hunter is judged on appearance conformation as well as performance.

"What do you think of her?" my friend asked.

I really didn't think much, but as we'd come so far I asked the dealer to have a rider put her over some jumps even though it was almost dark. One of the stable boys mounted her. Then the dealer said casually to another, "Hold out a stick, Tim."

Tim picked up a stick and held it horizontally about 4 feet above the ground. The rider put the mare at it and she jumped it easily.

Never in my life had I seen a horse that would jump a stick held in a man's hands. And the little mare had done it casually, without any careful approach or effort. When she jumped, she seemed to be flying. When she left the ground, she soared through the air, landing so gently that she gave the effect of floating down. And this in deep dusk when most horses would have had trouble even seeing a standard jump, let alone a thick stick held by a boy.

I said in a low voice to my friend, "Buy her!"

"Well, I don't know," he replied, pulling at his lip, "I don't think she's quite right for me."

I nearly slapped him. "Buy her!" I hissed between my teeth.

He looked at me, astonished. "Why, you don't even know her price!"

Controlling myself, I called to the dealer. "How much do you want for her?"

"Well, I'd have to get fifteen hundred to cover my expenses," he explained.

My friend shook his head. "I'll have to think that over."

While we drove back to Berwyn, my friend chattered about other things, scarcely mentioning the mare. I was going half out of my mind. I'd never dreamed a horse could jump like that. I wanted that mare more than I've ever wanted anything in my life. I knew she was worth far more than $1,500, even though at that time $1,500 might as well have been $15,000 as far as I was concerned. I didn't know what to do. I didn't think it would be honorable to buy the mare if my friend was really interested in her, yet if he wasn't, I was determined to get her before someone else could.

It was all I could do for the next few days to keep from demanding that my friend make up his mind and say definitely what he wanted to do. I forced myself to wait. Finally, he decided against getting her. Exactly ten seconds later I was on the telephone to the dealer. No, she hadn't been sold. I felt nearly sick with relief.

For the next few weeks, I was like a crazy person. It was summer so I was not attending classes and was relieved from my promise to the dean not to ride. In any case, I had forgotten all about veterinary school, my career, and everything else. I know that I frightened my parents and Norma. I started exercising horses at the Bel Air track and rode any animal they gave me. I rode some that even the professional riders wouldn't touch; big, savage brutes that were almost unmanageable. This went on for three weeks and every evening I'd call the dealer to make sure he hadn't sold my little mare—I already thought of her as "mine." Even so, it would take me weeks and weeks to make up her price.

Either Norma or Mother drove me to the track and then back home again while I lay in the back of the car so exhausted that I was only semi-conscious. Then one afternoon Father appeared at the track. I had just dismounted and was getting ready to get on another thoroughbred although my legs were trembling from weariness. Father said gently, "You won't need to do that now, Phyllis. Here's a check for fifteen hundred dollars so you can get the mare."

83

I clung to him crying and crying while he patted my shoulder. I knew he couldn't really afford the money and told him so. "I know I can't either," he agreed. "But Mother and I were afraid you were going to kill yourself." Still crying, I ran to the telephone and called the dealer. We clinched the deal over the phone, and as soon as I could get back to Berwyn and pick up a van, I was on my way to Dover.

The little mare's name was Cassadol. Our training—and love affair—together began immediately. As I've explained, a horse's eyes are so arranged that he cannot see an object a few feet in front. At the moment of jumping the animal jumps "blind," as it were, as it cannot see the top rail. To make sure that Cassadol didn't get too accustomed to a certain course, I used to van her to other people's courses to see how she'd do. I also traveled around to different shows, studying the various types of jumps and talking to the jump boys who set them up and repair them when a horse knocks one down. There are many kinds of jumps —in-and-out, post-and-rail, chicken coop, stone wall, brush, over water, and many, many more. I set out to learn the construction of each and how best to take it. The hardest jump for Cassadol was the straight up-and-down parallel pole jump. This is a double jump with a bar laid across two horizontal uprights and then, a few feet further on, a similar jump somewhat higher. The horse has to take both jumps at one bound. This is hard for any horse, but Cassadol was so little that as she came into it, the crossbar of the first jump hid the crossbar of the second. After a while she got to know that there would be a second bar there even if she couldn't see it.

Then, of course, she had to learn to come in on a certain lead when turning and approaching a jump. If she was on her left lead (leading with her left foreleg), I would have to balance to the left to steady her on the turn; if we were going clockwise, I would have to get her on the right lead. If for any reason she was on the wrong lead, I'd have to check her and shift my weight to put her on the right one.

In my experience, the last fence in a course is the greatest danger. In keen competition it is easy to forget the correct route around a course. The jumps are so arranged that they not only go around the edges but there are also some in the center and others at odd angles to test the horse's ability to turn and come in at awkward angles. You must follow a rigidly prescribed route and if you deviate from it by even one jump, you are immediately disqualified. I always go around the course on foot first and make up some silly jingle or other to help me memorize the correct pattern. Timing is crucially important. Often the rider who completes the course in the shortest possible time with the fewest faults wins, but one does not dare to go too fast. For example, when coming into the in-and-out—a boxlike set-up you must jump into and then out of—you can't go in too fast or the horse will pick up too much momentum and when he lands won't be able to get his legs under him for the out-jump. Then when you come to a spread jump—which is not so much a matter of height as length—the horse must be going close to his top speed to carry him across it, as with a person doing a broad jump.

The worst jumping is in the rain. The ground is slippery and when you take your turns, you can easily go down even with the most sure-footed horse. I've known the rain so bad I couldn't see the first rail of an oncoming jump. In such cases, I trusted Cassadol's instincts rather than my own.

There are a number of artificial ways of affecting a horse's jumping style, especially in "touch-and-out" classes, when a horse is disqualified if he touches a rail while going over it, even if he doesn't knock it down. These "touch-and-out" horses are pretty much a class of their own, as most jumpers—especially working hunters—will deliberately touch a fence with their feet to make sure where the rail is and steady themselves. This is not usually regarded as a fault but a virtue. There are common methods of forcing horses to lift their legs clear: they may be "poled," that is, a man stands by the jump and lashes them across the fetlocks as they go over. In another method a strand of catgut is stretched an inch or so higher than the rail. The horse cannot see this transparent strand and unless he keeps his hoofs up, will trip and have a painful fall. Some trainers put spiked boots on a horse's forelegs so that if he hits the rail, the spikes prick him. Others employ carpet strips—lengths cut from an old piece of carpet and studded with short nails—fastened to the top bar.

Not only are all these methods cruel and illegal; I personally think they are harmful. They make a horse fear the jumps. He never knows what will happen to him as he goes over, except that he soon learns it will be something painful. As a result, he will often refuse, jump unnecessarily high (which tires him and makes him land awkwardly), or become so unmanageable there's no handling him. To overcome these faults, some riders employ "charged" spurs—spurs with electric batteries in them that give the horse a severe shock if he refuses to go on. I've seen horses so tortured try to go straight up the wall of a building. Charged spurs are illegal even for training, although I've actually seen them used in shows. What the judges must have been thinking of to ignore them, I can't imagine.

There was never any question of any of these devices being used with dear little Cassadol. A horse that has to be electrically shocked before he'll perform isn't worth keeping, and the ill treatment is bound to show up in his performance sooner or later. Still, some professional riders will buy cheap horses that have either been ruined by stupidity or bad treatment, or else weren't really any good to begin with, and will try various drugs and mechanical tricks to make them win at a few shows so they can be sold for fancy prices. It is a terrifying feeling to be in a ring with one of these men and his half-mad mount, as you never know what either of them is going to do.

I started entering Cassadol in small shows where there was a stake class of $25 or $50, as money was terribly important to me at that time. She was really too small, I felt at first, to compete with the top open jumping horses, but as long as the competition was not too formidable, she could more than hold her own. Then I decided to take a big chance. I entered Cassadol in the famous Open Jumping Class at the Devon Horse Show, one of the big events in the East. I looked over the other horses and there was none I didn't think Cassadol could beat.

The Open Jumping Class was the first class of the evening. It was a time class; the fastest horse with the fewest number of faults would win. Several horses did very well but they had at least one fault and, as I was timing them, I knew Cassadol was faster. I patted her neck and told her we were going to win. She whinnied and turned around to press her soft nose against me as she always did when happy.

Suddenly through the gate came a big palomino, 17 hands high, ridden by one of the most famous professional riders in America. He moved with a power and grace I'd never seen before and it was obvious his rider knew exactly how to get the most out of him. He was much bigger than Cassadol, obviously stronger, and unquestionably faster.

"What horse is that?" I asked a groom who was standing near.

"Haven't you heard about him? I thought everyone had. That's Injun Joe, one of the great horses of all time. He's been selected by the Olympic Team and goes abroad in a couple of weeks. He's beaten just about every horse in the country in open jumping and he's a shoo-in to win the Olympics. I've got a hundred bucks riding on him and I wish it was a hundred thousand."

Injun Joe was indeed a great horse, who was to go on and win the Olympics. His name was changed to Nautical, and Walt Disney made a famous motion picture about him called *Nautical, the Horse with the Flying Tail*. I watched unbelievingly while the mighty palomino swept easily around the course. No faults on him, a perfectly clean round. At the finish the voice boomed over the loudspeaker: "No faults. Thirty-nine seconds."

Well, that took some beating. Cassadol and I were next. I knew the ring well and was able to give my little mare every advantage. She took the jumps like a bird, never faltering, never making a misstep. I cut all the corners I could, so even if she didn't have the big palomino's long stride, she made up for it in having a shorter distance to travel. When it was over, breathlessly I slid off her back and stood patting her neck, waiting for the verdict. It was not long in coming: "No faults." A pause. Then: "Thirty-nine seconds."

A tie: we would have to jump off. Cassadol was a little tired, while the powerful Injun Joe was still going strong. It would be a very close thing. I hoped Injun Joe would go first and give her a little longer to rest, but it was not to be. We were the first around.

No doubt about it, Cassadol was tiring. I carefully checked her curb, irons, and girth. Then we were off. I spoke to her softly and she put out her last burst of energy. We had a perfect round and I slid off, gave her a hug, and started walking her, for she was very hot. I told her I didn't care what happened, she had done perfectly, and if the bigger horse beat us it wasn't our fault. The loudspeaker announced: "No faults. Time thirty-eight seconds."

We had bettered our former time by one whole second. Now I could hear the thunder of the big palomino's hoofs as he pounded around the course. As he took each fence, a gasp went up from the crowd. What a powerhouse he was! Again he had a perfect round and his rider drew him in by the stands.

The loudspeaker clicked and then bellowed: "No faults! Thirty-eight seconds."

Another tie. That meant another jump-off. Only Cassadol wasn't up to it. I would have to concede.

Then the loudspeaker went on again: "—and one half second," it concluded.

We had won the great Devon Open Jumping Class against the most famous horse in America. The family came running out to me. I had my arms around Cassadol's neck and was crying. Father said, "Well, do you think she was worth fifteen hundred? We can always take her back." Mother and Norma were kissing me and Cassadol and sniffling. We had a victory supper on the tailgate of our station wagon afterwards. Cassadol got her favorite tidbit, an ice cream cone, for her share. I remember it was exactly seven o'clock on a Thursday night.

After that, I was convinced that Cassadol was unbeatable. The biggest show east of the Mississippi was coming up in the New York Armory and I entered Cassadol. This was quite a different affair from the Devon, important as Devon is. Devon is largely a social affair and although most of the riders are amateurs, some of the very top riders are career riders. The Armory show is highly professional. Tough, sometimes unscrupulous riders would be there, whose careers depended on their winning. The value of the horses would run into the millions.

The whole family went along. We rented a special trailer for the occasion, a great big thing so heavy that Father's little black Ford could hardly pull it. We had to leave long before dawn and the sun was just coming up when we started to enter the Lincoln Tunnel.

Mother had a map of the city and she acted as guide until we finally found the Armory. There had been a heavy snowfall a few days before, followed by a sudden thaw, and the streets were running rivers; the water must have been 10 inches deep and in many places was over the curb. We drove around the Armory but there didn't seem to be any way to get into the place. It was almost time for my first class and I was half-crazy. Then the Ford stalled.

I never knew there were so many cars in the world as the collection that piled up behind us—and all of them had horns. At last I got out, waded through the torrent in my good riding boots, got into the trailer, and tacked up Cassadol there. Then I backed her down the tailboard into the flood with dozens of cars honking at us and scores of men yelling curses. I was all prepared for the mare to bolt as no horse in the world could stand the racket plus the sudden descent into the deep water, and open jumpers are traditionally highly nervous, temperamental animals. But good little Cassadol never even flicked an ear. I led her through the rushing water and up on the sidewalk. This was my first encounter with New Yorkers and I must say it takes a good deal to surprise them. I know that I'd be surprised if I ran into a girl leading a horse down a sidewalk, but these people never even looked up. Cassadol kept her head on my shoulder for comfort and we forced our way through the crowd to the Armory. I finally found an open door and in we went. It was twenty minutes before our first class.

The Armory was gigantic; it took up a whole city block. The stands were packed and everyone seemed to be smoking. There was an army of horses. When our turn came, we went the course and Cassadol had only one fault, but there were six horses with no faults at all, so that was that. Meanwhile, the family had joined me. An officer had come up and ordered them to "get that thing out of there," to which Mother had replied, "I only wish we could." At last the officer had relented enough to call a tow truck and the Ford and trailer were now being overhauled in a garage. The garage was charging us $84, which seemed a fortune. Counting the entrance fee and our other expenses, Cassadol would have to get at least a third place for us to break even.

That afternoon was our second class: "touch-and-out." We touched and went out. Two failures. There was only one other class left and that was in the evening. It was the big event of the day: the Stake Class. First place meant $500 and national recognition. When we had started out that morning, I was more interested in the recognition. Now I was more interested in the money, for it would take me weeks of galloping horses around tracks to pay for this trip.

By five o'clock, the stands had emptied. I asked one of the ring boys where the people had all gone. He answered briefly, "Cocktail hour," and looked at me as though I were a hick from the sticks, which of course I was. I stayed with Cassadol as she was always nervous without me. We ate supper by the ring together; she got some grain from the trailer and I had a hot dog.

By eight-thirty the stands began filling up again although the Stake Class wasn't until ten-thirty. I watched the other trainers and riders getting ready. The Stake Class was a jumping event and they used poles, wires, and charged spurs on the horses. It was horrible to watch and I can't understand why it was allowed. The charged spurs were the worst. When the riders drove them home, the big horses—most of the 16 or 17 hands—literally went out of their minds. The trainers didn't seem to care; their jobs were at stake. Cassadol and I stood cowering in a remote part of the huge armory, watching the horror.

There were jumps down both sides of the ring and a triple bar jump in the center, one of the largest I'd ever seen, which was the hardest of all. On the first round, the jumps were 4 feet 6 inches. Dozens of horses took their turns and when it was over, there were eight clear, including Cassadol. The jumps were raised and we went around again. After three jump-offs, there were only two horses left, Cassadol and a giant gelding from Ohio, ridden by a well-known professional. By now, the noise in the place was deafening; yells, cheers, shouts, and boos. I kept talking to Cassadol and patting her as we got ready for the fourth jump-off. She was growing very tired. The triple jump had been raised to 5 feet 9 inches and the bars were spread further apart. To make it worse, the place was full of smoke. I know it sounds unbelievable but the smoke was so dense I couldn't see the top bar of the triple.

The other rider went first. He made a perfect round, then turned the great gelding toward the triple. I could see the horse's eyes gleam through the smoke. The gelding rose easily but I think not being able to see the top bar threw him off. He hit it full.

Then it was our turn. We also made a perfect round, although now the screams and yells were driving me mad and I knew they upset Cassadol. We turned toward the triple. I felt Cassadol gallop courageously and rise in the air, and as she went up, we came above the smoke and could see the top bar. She cleared it nicely. We'd won!

Cassadol was so hot I had to walk her around the ring until two-thirty that morning before I dared to load her. Then we started back. Both Father and Mother offered to drive but they were dead tired. I was beyond being tired. My eyes were frozen open and I felt like a machine that could go on and on. We got lost trying to get out of the city and found ourselves on the West Side Elevated Highway. Later, I learned that no trailers or trucks are allowed on it, but we didn't know that—all we knew was it pointed toward Philadelphia. At that hour there wasn't another car or a policeman in sight and we breezed along. Dawn came up as we went through Trenton and a few hours later we were home in Berwyn. Even then, it was a long time before I could relax and longer still before I could sleep.

It was Cassadol who made me well known in the horse world. Everyone thought I must be an expert to ride so well. The truth was that Cassadol did it all. She never made a mistake, although I often did. My main contribution to her training was love. I have never loved a horse—and I'm afraid few human beings—as I loved her.

I did get criticism from some professional riders. They thought I should push her more and use more of the standard methods for training a jumper. They did not realize that my little mare could not be pushed or punished and I refused to overwork her. She had so much spirit that abuse could easily have turned her into a dangerous animal. As it was, she loved to jump. She came into the ring eagerly, jumped her heart out, never refused a fence, and enjoyed the whole affair even more than I did. Fortunately, this came just at the right period for me as I had time enough to work her, travel with her, and groom her to perfection.

Once I thought that I was going to lose her. It was one of the most heartbreaking moments of my life.

I had entered her in the Open Jumping Class at Devon and as usual she had done magnificently and won the championship. All the newspapers were taking our picture and Father, standing behind the photographers, had a grin like a jack-o'-lantern; you could almost feel the happy glow that came from him. He had been boasting to his business friends about me and my wonderful mare and they had been politely skeptical. Well, when they opened the morning editions of their papers, they would see for themselves. After the photographers had finished, I was leading her to our van when a dealer came up to me.

"What do you want for her?" he asked.

"She's not for sale," I told him.

He took out his checkbook, signed his name to one of the checks, tore it out, and handed it to me. "Fill in the amount yourself," he said.

This is what in the horse world is called "an open check." I had heard of it but never seen it and never expected to as it is almost unknown. I stood staring at him.

"Suppose I filled it in for . . ." I hesitated, "thirty thousand dollars?"

He took the check back and I thought, *Well, that's that.* I wasn't surprised as I had purposely asked an absurd sum. But the dealer took out a pen and started filling in the check for the sum I'd asked.

"No, no!" I screamed. "She isn't for sale!" and I hurried her off to our van.

That night at the dinner table after my brother and sisters had left, I told Father and Mother about the dealer. For about half a minute they said nothing and I stopped breathing.

Then Father said slowly, "Phyllis, we're not rich people. That money would put you through veterinary school and set you up in practice. But let's look at it like this. If a stranger is willing to pay that much for Cassadol, what's she worth to us? No, she's your horse and you must keep her."

It isn't often I break down but I did then. Even so, it wasn't until years later that I realized what a sacrifice he and Mother were making and how much that money would have meant to them.

Cassadol was always a quicker thinker and steadier in the ring than I was. Once her quick thinking saved my life—or at least saved us both from a serious accident. Again, it was at Devon. That year there were fourteen horses in the jumping class and thirteen of them had gone around the course, none of them with a single fault. That gives you an idea of the competition we were up against, although at Devon the competition is always tough. I think it is the most demanding show in the East and possibly in the whole country. The jumping class was at night as usual as it is regarded as the climax of the week-long show. The ring was brilliantly lighted as Cassadol and I entered, the last entry of the show. I made my circle and headed Cassadol for the first jump. It was as dark as the bottom on an inkwell; no moon or stars, nothing but the golden ring surrounded by floodlights. Then as Cassadol got her haunches under her for the jump, the lights went out. Instantly we were in absolute darkness.

I was so startled I was paralyzed. I just sat there, unable to pull Cassadol in or make any motion. I think that any other horse in the world would have gone headlong into that jump—it was a high post-and-rail with heavy rails—and probably broken not only her neck but mine as well. Instead, Cassadol slid to a dead stop with her head almost touching the jump. At the same moment, I heard the cry of "Fire!" Now we had plenty of light for the stands were burning. There had been a short circuit. Sparks were spitting over the wooden bleachers and panic-stricken people were running for their lives.

I slid off and stood holding Cassadol's head. We were both shaking all over and I don't know which of us was the more scared. The crisis lasted only a few minutes. Then the short was corrected and the lights came on again.

The judges held a hasty conference and finally came over to me. "I hate to ask you to do this," a dignified older man explained. "But will you take another warm-up and try again? I know you're badly shaken and it's most unfair both to you and your mare, but the show is officially over tonight. Otherwise we would have to leave everything as it is until tomorrow and repeat the class. Many contestants are counting on leaving tonight and to postpone this final class would be a great hardship on everyone."

"We'll try it again," I told him.

Well, we only came third, but under the circumstances I think that was remarkable. No other horse could have done it.

Few people watching horse shows realize that what seems to be perfect form on the part of rider and steed is the result of innumerable minute details that have had to be foreseen and coordinated. Take just one example: shoeing. Each horse has to have shoes fitted in a slightly different way, and a rider has to be able to suggest to a blacksmith exactly how the horse is to be shod, based on the horse's stride and gait, and be there to supervise the shoeing. On top of that, the smith must be an expert craftsman and know quite a lot about a horse's anatomy. There was only one smith in whom I had complete trust, the strange old Irishman Willy Bradley. He always shod Cassadol and knew precisely how to do it. Even so, I always took pains to be there during the shoeing.

There was a very important show at York, Pennsylvania, where I wanted to exhibit Cassadol to win points for state championship. By bad luck, Willy was sick, so I had to get another blacksmith who was highly recommended. I spoke to the man over the telephone and asked him to do the shoeing, explaining that I positively did not want my mare shod unless I was there. He agreed.

When I came home the next day, Mother said casually, "Oh, Phyllis, the blacksmith was here and shod Cassadol so she's all ready for York." I was shocked and ran for the barn with Mother anxiously following me. Afraid of what I might find, I checked Cassadol's feet while Mother stood by. The front feet were fine but the rear shoes were not. Willy had always left a ridge on the inside of the shoes for the hind legs to give the mare better footing in wet weather, which was especially important with Cassadol as after a jump she landed running. This was wonderful for me as there was no jar; she just seemed to float along and was away again instantly without a pause, an important consideration when time was a factor. Still, if the course was slippery, it was a handicap as she was liable to slip or misstep unless specially shod.

"I know the man didn't shoe her like Willy Bradley," Mother said, worried that she had done wrong. "But he explained that she would move better this way."

So she probably would—if it didn't rain. I considered calling the smith back and telling him to change the hind shoes but that would mean more nail noles in Cassadol's little hoofs, so I decided to take the chance and hope for good weather.

As usual, the whole family went with us. The show lasted for three days. By the end of the second day, we were so far ahead on points that on the last day all we had to do was go around the course to win. Cassadol had never, but never, failed to complete a course, so the championship was as good as pinned on her. Then it started to rain.

And did it rain! It rained all night and all the next day. When the jumping class began that evening, it was still drizzling. We were last to compete or enter the ring again. I watched the other horses slipping and sliding but most of them made it around, although not one had a clean round; all ran up several faults. Then it was our turn.

Even though I had all the confidence in the world when it came to Cassadol, I couldn't believe the exhibition she put on. She took every fence clean. Finally, there were only two left. She took one clean as usual, then came down on turf slippery as grease. Her hind legs went out from under her and she tilted over on one side. I tried to kick my feet out of the stirrups and jump clear, but it was too late. She came down on top me, all four feet in the air, pinning my left leg under her. The pain was unbelievable. Then she rolled over on her other side. I know it sounds incredible, yet I have always believed she did it deliberately to free my leg. I managed to crawl clear. My leg was fractured although I didn't know it at the time. I was thinking only of Cassadol. Mud the size of a football was jammed under her saddle and I could tell that she'd hurt herself although just how badly I didn't know.

Men came running to our help. One of them shouted: "Get an ambulance!" for I was limping badly. "I don't need it!" I screamed at him. "I want to stay with my horse!"

I managed to get Cassadol on her feet. She had strained her rear left leg but luckily not badly. We limped out of the ring together and I got her into our van. I never allowed her to be put in a stall where another horse had been for fear she might pick up some infection as stalls in show stables often are not kept as clean as they might be. We made it home all right, but of course we were disqualified in the jumping class and it was many months before we could make up the points we'd lost. For the next six weeks, we were both laid up and barely able to walk. Mother and I bathed Cassadol's leg and rubbed it until it is a wonder we did not rub all the hair off. She healed completely, but it was a close thing.

I think my proudest moment with Cassadol was at the Bloomsburg Show in central Pennsylvania, given near my parents' home town. It was not the biggest show in the world nor the best but all our relatives were there. It was especially important to me because when I had first begun to show Cassadol a year before, we had competed in this show. My sister Norma had been in it then too, riding a saddlebred in the Walk, Trot, and Canter Class. Norma had done very well and got a ribbon. Everyone was very proud of her, as they should have been. Our relatives were rather simple country folk and when they heard that I, a young girl, was riding in the Open Jumper Class, they were shocked. "That's much too dangerous," Grandmother told my mother. "It isn't at all suitable for a woman, especially a girl. Why can't Phyllis ride in a gentle class like Norma?"

Mother replied that she had every confidence in me, so in spite of my relatives' doubts, I went ahead. Cassadol was a green jumper at that time and she was convinced it was her duty to jump everything in sight no matter how impossible. I was a green rider and did not know how to control her. Still, we did beautifully until we came to the in-and-out, the double jump with two horizonal bars supported by posts 24 feet apart.

Cassadol came charging up to the in-and-out in her best style. Not for her the slow method of taking the two jumps one at a time; she was determined to take the whole jump at one bound. We went flying up into the air and dear Cassadol did her best, but even a kangaroo can't jump 24 feet. We came crashing down on top of the second bar, all mixed up and in a dreadful state.

No, we did not win any ribbons that day. Grandmother remarked austerely: "Well, when that girl kills herself, don't say I didn't tell you so."

Fortunately nothing was hurt except our pride. Since that sad day, Cassadol and I had jumped many a jump and knew all about ins-and-outs. One year later, we returned to the Bloomsburg Show. Again all our relatives had turned out, including Grandmother, as disapproving as ever.

This time it was different. Everything went as smooth as Cassadol's stride and we won the championship. As the judge came over to pin us, Grandmother remarked triumphantly to Mother: "I knew all along that Phyllis could do it. Remember I told you so!"

I had Cassadol for fourteen years. She died one Thursday evening at seven o'clock: the exact day and hour that she'd beaten Nautical at Devon, her first great victory. I had her buried at our farm upcountry in a big oak box with all her tack. I have never seen another horse to equal her.

5

WOMAN HORSE DOCTOR

ELAINE HOPKINS AND I FINALLY GRADUATED FROM VETERINARY school in 1957. It was the climax of nine years of hard work but I only felt numb at the time. I was too exhausted by the final examinations. Then we had to take the state boards, three full days of the hardest sort of work. I remember the temperature was 90 degrees. My hands stuck to the papers so I could hardly write.

Then, at long last, it was all over. Elaine and I were licensed veterinarians. My family gave a big party for us to celebrate the great event.

In the middle of the celebration, the telephone rang and Father answered it. He came back looking a little peculiar. "Phyllis, it's A. A. Biddle on the phone." At that name, everyone stopped talking. Mr. Biddle was a fabulous figure. He was enormously wealthy, mad about horses, and owned one of the best stables in our part of the country. He was the head of the most prominent family on the Main Line. He was also famous for his eccentricities; some people frankly considered him a little mad. "He wants you to come over at once and check some of his mares to see if they are in foal."

Dr. Bartholomew had taught me the trick of palpating the uterus of a mare and I could tell eighteen days after she had been covered if she was in foal. It wasn't a method generally known at the time, although it was very accurate; most veterinarians had to wait seventy days before they could tell. If a mare hasn't "settled" after having been bred, she must be bred again as soon as possible otherwise the foal will be born too late in the year to compete with the older foals. Mr. Biddle had seen me checking mares at a stable with Dr. Bartholomew and had evidently been impressed by the technique and remembered me now that Dr. Bartholomew wasn't available.

"It's a great chance for you," said Father, although he still looked worried. "Mr. Biddle can be a good friend if he likes you. If he doesn't or thinks you've let him down—well, there'd be no use in your trying to practice in this part of the country. With him, it's always touch-and-out; one touch and you're out. This is your first case and you're still young and inexperienced. Do you want to try it?"

"Of course I do," I said. I couldn't understand why he was so worried.

"I'll go with you," promised Elaine.

Elaine drove, obviously thinking that I'd be too nervous. As it turned out, Elaine was the nervous one. Like everyone else who has had any connection with Philadelphia, she'd heard of the Biddles. They were as typically Philadelphian as scrapple, a special dish made of minced pork, herbs, corn, and other ingredients that has never caught on elsewhere, although no proper Philadelphian would dream of eating breakfast without it. There is a favorite story that when the Prince of Wales, later Edward VIII, visited Philadelphia, he gave a courteous speech on leaving, saying: "I have so greatly enjoyed eating your famous breakfast food, the Biddles, and wish to thank the Scrapples for their generous hospitality." It really made no difference, as the Biddles and scrapple are equally Philadelphian.

Even I was cowed when Elaine turned into the entrance of the Biddles' 200-acre estate near Newtown Square. This was the heart of the horse country in those days. Newtown Square itself was a tiny village surrounded by vast breeding farms. We drove up a lane lined by great sugar maples whose branches joined hands over our heads. We had to drive slowly as every few yards there was a "thank-you ma'am" across the road: a raised strip of concrete that forced you to come to a stop and ease the car over it if you didn't want a broken spring.

Soon we came upon a series of warning signs. The first one read: "Drive slowly! Deaf Dog!" That's one I'll never forget. It was followed by others: "Beware! Duck Crossing!" "Valuable Chickens! Proceed with caution!" Elaine inched along, keeping a lookout for the dozens of dogs, ducks, chickens, and geese that were all over the place.

We finally came to an old, rambling Victorian Gothic mansion. Behind it were the stables, the largest and most elaborate I'd ever seen. Mr. Biddle himself came out to meet us. He was a big man, rather heavy, in his early sixties, with gray hair just beginning to recede. He was handsome, and although soft-spoken, he was not the kind of a man I'd care to offend. He wielded tremendous power and knew it. He was responsible to no one and did not expect anything he said to be questioned.

Elaine and I got out of the car, I carrying my brand-new veterinarian's bag. We were both in spotless white coveralls and had made sure our boots were shined. He looked us over and I had an uneasy feeling that the newness of everything made him suspicious.

He cleared his throat. "Ah, how many pregnancies have you examined in your career, young lady?" he asked pleasantly, but looking at me sharply from under bushy eyebrows.

"Oh, twenty-five or thirty," I answered lightly. This wasn't really a lie. I had checked at least that many mares. I only omitted to say that Dr. Bartholomew had always been there with me, giving me instructions and checking my results.

Mr. Biddle stood looking at me expressionlessly for a few seconds. I stood looking back at him. This was one veterinarian job I knew I could do well; probably better than anyone else, due to Dr. Bartholomew's months of instruction. At last Mr. Biddle turned and led the way to the stables.

He had seventeen horses at this time, all thoroughbreds and several well known on the track. Each animal was in a spacious box stall with a sliding wooden door fitted with a line of black iron bars so every detail of the stall was plainly visible to anyone walking down the aisle. Each stall had its own window and in addition there were skylights set in the ceiling so that the stables were almost as light as outside. The name of each horse was printed in large letters on a blackboard fastened to the door. We passed the tackroom where the reins, bits, saddles, and so on were kept. It had wall-to-wall carpeting and was cleaner than most parlors. The tack was hung on wooden pegs and kept behind glass so dust would not injure it. We saw stablemen putting down fresh, golden straw and removing any that had been fouled. The stables smelled wonderfully of straw, hay, oats, and the clean, invigorating odor of horses in perfect condition.

Mr. Biddle stopped. "These mares were covered three weeks ago," he said, indicating a line of stalls. "There are eight of them and it is important that I know immediately if they have settled. I have spoken to several other vets and they tell me they would have to wait for forty-five days. That's too long for me. I must know now and I must know accurately. Do you understand?"

"Yes, I can tell you now and I will be one hundred percent correct," I said confidently. I saw Elaine shudder at my boldness.

I pulled on a polyethylene sleeve and felt inside the first mare while a groom held her head. I had had so much practice at this delicate work, I could tell if the embryo was in the left or right horn of the uterus, its size, and if it was too soft or too hard. I was able to tell Mr. Biddle that all but two of the mares had settled. "I'd like to come back in forty-five days and check again to make sure everything is going all right," I added.

He said that would be splendid. He seemed pleased with me. Just then a curious-looking chicken entered the stable and stood watching us in a way that made me nervous. Mr. Biddle pointed to it. "That is one of my most valuable chickens. A very rare breed. I wouldn't sell it for any amount of money." I tried to look impressed although I thought it was the stupidest-looking creature I'd ever seen, but then I'm not an expert on chickens. Before we left, Mr. Biddle asked, "Will you two young ladies come over to the cow barn? I have something I'd like you to see."

We followed him to a barn some distance away. There in a stall was a wretched-looking steer, sweating profusely and walking around and around in a circle. "Have you any idea what's wrong with him?" Mr. Biddle asked me.

"Yes," I said confidently. "He has listeriosis." Actually, I had never seen an animal suffering from this ailment, but I'd read about it. The symptoms were unmistakable.

Mr. Biddle suddenly whirled on me. "You seem to know a surprising amount for someone just starting practice. Well, the bovine vet is coming tomorrow. I'll see if you're putting up a bluff. I don't like people who put up bluffs," and he abruptly walked away.

Elaine and I were stunned at this rudeness. In silence we returned to the horse barn. Everything was so neat there that I was determined to leave it exactly as I'd found it so there would be no cause for complaint. I took my used polyethylene sleeve with me instead of discarding it as I would ordinarily have done, emptied the stainless-steel bucket by throwing the dirty water plus disinfectants out the door, and cleaned everything up perfectly. When we left, I took the wheel with Elaine sitting strangely silent beside me. "I really think everything went perfectly," I said somewhat smugly. "I wouldn't be surprised if Mr. Biddle lets me take over his whole stables. Not a single hitch."

"Just one," said Elaine. She sounded grim.

I felt as though someone had just kicked me in the stomach. "What do you mean?"

Reaching under her coat, Elaine produced the dead body of Mr. Biddle's prize chicken. "When you threw out that bucket of hot water, you hit him. He must have had a weak heart, for he dropped dead."

I sat staring at the dead chicken as though it had been a human corpse. "I'll never make it in practice," I gasped. "I'm ruined!"

"No you're not," said Elaine. "I grabbed the chicken right away and hid him. No one will ever know."

And no one has—until now. It's been a secret Elaine and I have carried in our hearts all these years. Thank heaven I can now confess and get it off my conscience. I've always felt gulity about murdering that poor chicken.

On the way home, I also worried over the steer. I was certain he must have listeriosis, yet it was obvious from Mr. Biddle's manner that if I'd made a mistake, he was through with me. Perhaps luckily, I soon had something else to think about. We encountered one of those terrible thunderstorms that seem peculiar to the Delaware Valley. Neither Elaine nor I usually mind thunderstorms but this was really frightening. Lightning was all around us and the explosions of thunder seemed to lift the car off the road. Gradually the storm passed, leaving behind the signs of its rage: trees with broken limbs, power lines down, and judging from the distant wail of fire sirens, more than one burning building.

When we finally made it home, we found my family had delayed dinner for us. In spite of my guilty conscience over Mr. Biddle's prize chicken and my fears for the steer, I was ravenously hungry. All during the long period of studying for exams I had been unable to eat; even drinking a cup of coffee nauseated me. Now I intended to make up for it.

Mother instantly put our steaks on the grill. Mother is an expert at picking out savory steaks and the smell of these was maddening; the choicest cuts, with just enough fat to give them flavor. Usually I liked my steaks rather well done, only this time I was too hungry to wait. The meat was still rare when I put it on my plate and cut off a large slice—then the phone rang. Father answered it.

He returned looking unhappy. Mother said, "Oh, no—not again!"

"It's some man who lives a couple of miles from here. His children have a pony, a little mare, and she was just due to foal. They had her out in the pasture and she's been struck by lightning. She's dead but he thinks Phyllis may be able to save the foal if she hurries."

"Couldn't they get someone else?" Mother asked. "Phyllis has had a hard two weeks, a hard day, and she's half-starved."

"No one else could get there in time."

I put down my fork and looked sadly at the steak. "At any rate, it will be here when I get back," I said, getting up. "Where's my bag?"

"Do you mind if I don't come this time?" asked Elaine unhappily. "I'm awfully hungry."

"Just don't eat my steak too," I warned her as I headed for the car.

Father had gotten good directions. It was still raining and the road was slippery, but I knew every second was important and went as fast as I could. Soon I saw a man standing, holding open a gate, and waving me in excitedly.

"Where's the mare?" I shouted, as my car skidded in the wet mud.

"Under that tree. It's the only tree in the pasture," he yelled back.

I could just see the tree. It had obviously been struck by lightning and the pony had been standing under it to get out of the rain. I went at top speed across the grass and mud, constantly fearful that the car would mire down. As I pulled up beside the tree, I could see the dead mare and all around her, seared, burnt grass. She had a great burn right across her body, straight as a girth.

I jumped out of the car before it had stopped moving, scalpel in hand. The mare was fat, very fat indeed, as was to be expected in the last few days of pregnancy. I cut carefully through the layers of yellow tissue, taking great precautions not to injure the foal. It was unpleasant work because the smell of the burnt flesh was overpowering. I opened the womb: there was nothing there.

The man arrived in a tractor with five little children. They were screaming anxiously, "Where's our baby pony?"

I had to tell them the truth, whereupon they all burst into tears. I felt like crying myself. I also had an uneasy feeling that I was going to be sick. The stench of the roasted horse, the fact that I was dropping with exhaustion and hadn't eaten anything for what seemed to be days, added to my problem. Then I found that my car was stuck in the mud. The farmer had to pull me out with his tractor.

I drove home wishing that in some way I'd been able to produce a foal for the sobbing children, even if I'd smuggled it in under my coveralls. Clearly all that had consoled them for the loss of their pet was the prospect of having her foal. There was nothing I could do. The mare had gorged herself on the rich pasture grass and the family had confused her plumpness with pregnancy.

At home, everyone else had finished eating. As I sat down at the table, Mother proudly put a well-done steak under my nose. I took one whiff and that was that. I was sick at last, good and sick, and Mother and Norma had to put me to bed.

Mr. Biddle had been so abrupt with me over the matter of the steer that I didn't expect to hear from him again. Then, a few days later, a box arrived with two dozen lovely long-stemmed roses. Frankly, I'm not all that used to getting flowers, especially long-stemmed roses. I opened the card in amazement. It was from Mr. Biddle. I read: "The steer did have listeriosis. I beg your pardon for doubting you. I hope you will forgive me—and also take over my stables."

I forgave him.

Vetting the Biddle stables was a great honor but no sinecure. Mr. Biddle never interfered with me, never followed me about asking questions, never questioned my judgment, but he never missed a trick. He always required me to come to his luxurious living room after I had examined his horses and report on the condition of each animal. I was given a book in which each horse had a separate page. I had to write up the animal's condition on his page, then I would report to Mr. Biddle and read him my findings. Usually I went to his stable first thing in the morning, as he always served breakfast. Ham, eggs, bacon, and of course scrapple and the strongest coffee I've ever encountered.

Some days I was grateful for such a delicious meal. Other times, when I was in a hurry to get to my next appointment, it was a nuisance to have to sit there and eat, especially if I didn't feel hungry, but none of this made any difference to Mr. Biddle. When he ate, everyone ate. The meal was served, not by a butler or a waitress in uniform, but by a Ukrainian woman who wore sacks around her feet instead of shoes. While we ate, Mr. Biddle would rise occasionally and study a ticker tape installed in the living room. He would then call his office and say something like, "Buy fifty thousand shares of MX & W." Having your own private ticker tape in your home struck me as the height of luxury.

Mr. Biddle was a widower. He had a life-sized portrait of his wife hanging in the hallway and often used to stand looking at it and, I think, talking to it, although I never saw his lips move. He was fond of women and many came to see him, yet it was clear that they meant nothing to him. I'm sure his wife was the only woman he ever loved.

He had two grown daughters and a son who lived with him,

but as my work was confined entirely to the horses I seldom saw them. Mr. Biddle was a whimsical man. Sometimes everyone in the household had to speak only French; at other times, he went on strange diets. On occasion, he would sit and play the guitar for hours. He played very well, too. Sometimes during our meals, he would tell me stories of his travels, especially in England and Hungary. What he was doing in Hungary, I never knew, but he surely loved the country. During the mornings he never touched a drop of liquor, then at two o'clock he would start to drink. It was incredible the amount he could put away, but I never saw it affect either his speech or movements. It did, however, hit him in another curious fashion.

In the hallway he kept a large table covered with various sorts of hats: top hats, deerstalkers, driving caps, derbies, straw hats, and so on. After a few drinks he would go to the table, select one of the hats, and put it on. For the rest of the day he would be whatever character the hat implied. If it were a workman's hat, he would hitch up his trousers, say a few words in a coarse, ungrammatical manner, and go out on the grounds to do some manual work. If he decided on the top hat, he would instantly become a polished, elegant gentleman making polite conversation and asking me if I intended to attend the Assembly this year. It was an innocent hobby and caused me trouble only on one occasion.

I had to check fifteen mares at this time and they were out in the pasture. They were quite tame and I could handle them easily, so rather than bother the grooms, I went out to examine them in the field. Mr. Biddle passed me wearing the deerstalker hat and carrying a shotgun, every inch the country gentleman. He was headed for a lake, where there was a flock of mallard ducks.

I had just begun to examine the first mare when *bang!*—a shot went off seemingly in my ear. I went straight up in the air and the mare took off across the field as though she were running in the Grand National. After considerable trouble, I managed to get hold of her again and *bang!*—another shot boomed out and off she went again. After a while, I gave up and got the grooms to help me, but even so it was more like a rodeo than an ordinary examination. When I finally finished, I wrote up my report and went looking for Mr. Biddle. He was sitting in the library, still wearing the deerstalker.

"Nothin' like a bit of sport, eh?" he said with a pronounced English accent as I came in. "Jolly good shootin'. Sorry you missed it."

I only wished that I had missed it, but I read him my report while he nodded his head and asked me some very penetrating questions, for he did know a great deal about horses. When I had finished, he accompanied me to my car. Norma and I had spent a large part of that morning cleaning out the interior, which I had allowed to get messy, as I'd been too busy that week to worry about it. I hate housework of any kind, and scrubbing leather seats, vacuuming floors, and polishing windows seemed a terrible drag. I never would have finished if it hadn't been for Norma's help, but now the inside of the car was immaculate and I regarded it proudly.

"I say, one moment if you don't mind," exclaimed Mr. Biddle, and hurried off. I did mind as I was already late for my next appointment, but I waited. In a few minutes Mr. Biddle returned with a string of the deadest ducks I've ever seen. Most of them were blown into bloody fragments, bits and pieces hanging by sinews, feathers falling off at every step he took. Casually, Mr. Biddle tossed the gory mess into the back of my nice clean car.

"Nothin' like a bit of game," he assured me. "Serve them with bacon strips, sage, and salt and pepper to taste. No, no!" He held up a warning hand. "No thanks! Glad to be of service. Well, tally-ho and all that." It took Norma and me most of the evening to get the car clean again. I gave the ducks a decent burial.

I worked with Mr. Biddle for many years. He was one of the last of the old Main Line stock. Men like him don't exist any more, which is sad. The world is poorer for their passing.

For much longer than I care to remember, Mr. Biddle was virtually my only client. It wasn't easy for a young veterinarian, especially a girl, to find people who would entrust their valuable animals to her. I'm not especially good with small animals and everyone seemed to expect a woman veterinarian to specialize in them; as a matter of fact, the few veterinarians who were women usually did. I was still waiting hopefully for another stable when a hair stylist and his wife came to me to have the dewclaws of their pet poodle removed.

Dogs often have trouble with elongated or infected dewclaws, and I had performed this extremely simple operation several times. It can hardly be called an operation; there is really nothing to it. I would have been hesitant about my ability to perform many operations on a dog, but I most certainly could remove dewclaws.

The couple were at the same time touching and a little ridiculous. Both were immaculately groomed. The woman had every hair on her head lacquered in place; her magnificent gown seemed to have been lacquered on also. She wore enormous earrings and stage makeup. Her husband had a ruffled shirt front, a carefully designed hairdo, which he had to repair with a small comb from time to time, several rings on his slender manicured hands, and a mustache that was hardly thicker than his wife's painted eyebrows. The poodle was equally a work of art. He was a prizewinner and they proudly told me what he had cost as a puppy. I forget the sum, but it left me stunned. You could have bought a racehorse for the amount. He was wearing a specially designed collar and a fur coat conceived and made by his owner. I should get to wear such a coat! In spite of all this splendor, he was a miserably nervous little animal who had obviously never been allowed to run about or play with other dogs. When I picked him up, he trembled convulsively in my arms while I tried to quiet him.

His master and mistress would not stay. As they departed, holding each other's hands for comfort, the woman turned to me and said, "We've never been able to have children. We've tried to adopt a baby but all the agencies have turned us down. Tootsie is our only baby. Take care of her." Her eyes were moist as they hurried out.

Between Tootsie's convulsive shaking and this tragic speech, I was feeling a trifle nervous myself. I decided to get the operation over with quickly. I put a muzzle on Tootsie to prevent her biting, if she felt inclined to do so (this is a standard precaution in operations even of the most minor kind), and prepared to remove the troublesome dewclaws. Suddenly Tootsie aspirated, or to put it more simply, she vomited. Because of the muzzle, the vomit went into her lungs. She gave an agonized jerk, then became limp.

I grabbed a scalpel and cut the muzzle off. Tootsie still hung lifeless. Not daring to believe what I now knew to be the truth, I put a stethoscope to her chest. Her heart had stopped beating.

Looking back, I can recall two terrible moments in my life and I do not know which was the worst. The first was when that half-broken colt dragged me around the track by one leg. This was the second. I came closer to panic than I ever have before or since. I knew well what the little poodle's death would mean to her owners. For a moment, I lost my head. I grabbed the dead dog by the hind legs and shook her insanely, crying, "You can't die! You can't die!" It was a pointless action. There was no motive, no good reason for it. Yet a miracle happened. As I shook the dog, the vomit choking her was dislodged and poured out. I heard Tootsie give a gasp and then open her eyes. I put her on the operating table and massaged her heart until she recovered.

It was only several hours later that I could bring myself to remove the dewclaws, and naturally I did not muzzle her again; I got Norma to hold her head. The couple returned, congratulated me on doing such an expert job, and departed with a happy, lively Tootsie. That happened many years ago, but the memory of the fright I got is still painful.

As vetting the Biddle stable only took a comparatively short time, I had to find other clients. After my experience with Tootsie, I looked around for larger animals. Finally I found a woman living by herself on a big farm north of Doylestown—which in those days really meant out in the boondocks—who had a herd of dairy cattle and needed a veterinarian. This woman had never been able to get along with a male veterinarian. I soon found out why.

The woman, or I should say "lady" as she belonged to a prominent Main Line family I shall call the Straffords, was a curious personality both physically and mentally. Miss Strafford was big, not fat; simply a Brünhilde: tall, well proportioned, and amazingly powerful. I have known few men as strong as she was. She was in her early twenties and had attended the most exclusive schools, although they did not seem to have left much of an impression on her. Miss Strafford had quarreled with her parents and bought this isolated farm where she lived completely alone. She did all the work herself.

The house was Colonial, parts of it going back to the seventeenth century. It was approached by a long drive lined with dogwoods that were like a vision of paradise in spring; you seemed to be driving between perfumed snowbanks. By the front door there was a stone mounting block where in former years ladies and gentlemen had mounted their horses for the hunt. The beams and mantlepiece were of wood but had been "marbled" in some forgotten era by dipping a feather in paint and stroking them to imitate the bluish pattern of marble. There was a brick foyer, a fireplace big enough to roast a whole sheep, and deep window ledges.

The barn was kept immaculate. It was a very old barn, perhaps even older than the house. The overhang was so low it resembled a tunnel. Inside, the old beams had rotted or given way and the loft was supported by iron girders. It was so low I could reach up and touch the roof. I remember that she had to lock on the covers of the trash cans to keep out the raccoons. Around the barnyard was a stone wall covered with ivy and roses. It was all cobblestoned. Miss Strafford had a small flock of guinea fowl that acted as watchdogs and always set up a shrill rattling cry when anyone came on the property. They nested at night in a single apple tree that grew up in the center of the barnyard from a hole among the cobbles.

I soon found out that to handle cattle successfully, you must be around them and know how they behave. I was first called in on the routine task of inoculating the herd and putting on ear tags. Miss Strafford had the animals in the barnyard, but unfortunately it had been raining and the cobbles were covered with manure and mud. She indicated the herd with a wave of her hand. "There they are, go right ahead," and left me.

If I had been older and more experienced I would never have tried to inoculate twenty head of cattle by myself. I tried lassoing them, one after another. I could get the lasso on; the question was what to do after that. The cows were much stronger than I was and dragged me through the mud, hanging onto the end of the rope. They especially disliked having the ear tags clamped on—it must have been really painful. I was still only half through the job with my coveralls ruined and so exhausted I could hardly stand when my Brünhilde happened to walk past carrying a bucket of sweetfeed. She stopped amazed.

"How did you get yourself so dirty?" she demanded. I told her from wrestling a herd of infuriated cattle.

"Why, they're only cows." She did not speak contemptuously but simply stated a fact. "Anyone can handle cows. Here, I'll show you." She put down the bucket, walked into the barnyard, went over to the nearest cow, and grabbed it by the nose. The cow struggled but she had a grip on its nostrils like a T-clamp. In seconds the cow realized that it had met its mistress and stood still while I inoculated it and put on the ear tag.

"I'd better help you," said Miss Strafford, in her matter-of-fact way. "You were foolish not to have called on me before. It never occurred to me you might be having trouble with such easy creatures as cows." Just then, a particularly mean animal charged her with horns lowered. Casually she reached out, grabbed one horn, bulldogged it, then clamped on her nose grip while I hurriedly filled my hypodermic. "No hurry, no hurry," she remarked, while the raging cow ducked and plunged, trying to gore her. "Do you know, I think you've taken up the wrong line of work. You're too small and delicate to be a veterinarian. I'd advise you to switch to some other profession."

There was nothing abusive in her tone or manner; she was just being frank. Miss Strafford also gave me several useful hints on how to handle cattle and then went on to tell me how to give injections. Now it so happens that I am quite good at giving injections; it was one of the techniques Dr. Charles taught me. Without raising my voice or losing my temper, I showed her why I gave them the way I did. She watched closely, asked a few questions, then remarked, "Yes, I see now." Never again did she criticize my technique in this respect, although when she felt I was doing something wrong, she always told me bluntly what it was.

I could understand why Miss Strafford had never gotten along with male veterinarians. No man would stand having a woman tell him what to do, especially a woman with no medical background. Actually, Miss Strafford knew a great deal about cows. When foot rot developed in the herd, she showed me how to tie a rope around a cow's leg, throw the rope over a beam, then lift the leg so the animal was immobile. I would never have thought of it myself because if you tried such a stunt with a horse, he'd thrash himself to death. With the animal helpless, treating foot rot was a simple business. You only had to cut out the infection and then pack the hoof. It cured itself.

A much worse job was freeing a retained placenta. With cows, the placenta is "buttoned" onto caruncles attached to the uterus, unlike mares, whose placentas readily separate from the endometrium. There are advantages and disadvantages both ways. A cow is far less likely to abort than a mare, but if after the calf has been born the placenta is not discharged, as soon as the blood ceases to circulate through it, the placenta rots. This will eventually prove fatal to the cow.

Knowledgeable as Miss Strafford was about cattle, she had neglected to look for the placenta after one of the cows calved, nor did she notice that the mother was listless and running a high fever. It was three days later before she finally called me. As soon as I saw the cow, I knew what was wrong. The smell alone was diagnostic to me. It would be a tricky business because while peeling the placenta free, it was easy to tear the delicate lining of the uterus. That would cause hemorrhaging and certain death.

I went to work while Miss Strafford held the tortured animal's head. The stench was so bad I thought I would faint. I used antiseptics by the bucketful, mainly to counteract the awful odor, with plenty of water. Each of the little caruncles had to be freed while I pressed my forehead against the cow's rump and tried to hold my breath. When the placenta finally came away, I reeled out into the barnyard to recover. It required days to get rid of the stink. It was worse than the skunk.

I took care of this remarkable lady's cows for ten years. She loved certain of her cows and treated them like pets. Even though she was extremely opinionated, she would always listen to reason. After she told me what to do, if I replied, "Well, I do it differently," she would ask in her usual blunt way, "Why?" I would always explain in detail while she listened. If she was convinced that I was right, there was never another word said on the subject. Sometimes she *was* right, especially in matters concerning the handling of the stock.

During my first year as a veterinarian, I also took over a flock of eighty-five sheep. They were pedigreed Cheviot and were owned by a wealthy family who kept them as a hobby. The family also employed a full-time shepherd who had nothing to do except during lambing time. That was a busy season for both of us, as I had to attend every birth no matter what the hour or the condition of the roads. I had originally been called in to treat the old ram, a gigantic animal nearly as big as a pony. He was sick and dispirited, but try as I would I could find nothing wrong with him. Then by chance I ran my hand along one of his long, curved horns and found that it was growing back into his head. With the shepherd's help, I was able to cut off the tip although the ram put up a terrible battle which, after all, was understandable. The family were so impressed that they took me on as the flock's veterinarian. As I needed the money, I was delighted.

Aside from lambing, my only real duty was to worm the flock. I did this for several years, then it occurred to me that it was rather ridiculous for me to be paid a good round fee to do something that the shepherd could do just as well. I suggested to the family that I show the shepherd what to do, and they agreed. I gave the man a gallon of worm medicine, explaining how to measure the correct dosage, and left convinced that everything would go well.

The next day, I got a call from the family. Half the flock were down and five were dead. I rushed to the farm. There was no doubt about it; the sheep were suffering from worm medicine poisoning. With emetics, I was able to save the rest, but I couldn't understand what had happened. Had the batch of medicine I'd given him been bad or was there some other explanation?

"You didn't overdose them, did you?" I asked the man.

"No, sir, Doctor. I was careful only to give them what you said. Here's the cup I used to measure out the dose."

He handed me a graduate marked for both cubic centimeters and ounces. He had used the wrong scale. Someone who is used to handling drugs and measuring dosages does not realize that the average person can make mistakes in even the simplest matters. I never forgot that lesson—but it didn't bring back the five pedigreed sheep.

For a long time it seemed as though Mr. Biddle was going to be the only horse owner who had faith in me. I was called in occasionally but only when no male veterinarian was available. Then I got my second break.

A Colonel Robert Dale called. It sounded like the same old deal. He had a valuable stallion who was to breed a mare that day and he wanted me to wash up the stud to make sure the mare did not receive any infection, a routine breeding procedure. There are professional ethics among veterinarians, so I asked him, "Why doesn't your regular veterinarian do it?" expecting to hear that the man was sick or unavailable.

Back came the surprising answer: "He's afraid of the animal. This stud is a killer and my vet won't go near him."

"Why did you happen to select me?"

The colonel was frank. "Because I've heard you're crazy and will try anything."

Naturally, I had to live up to this tribute. "I'll be right over," I assured him. I didn't tell the family anything, as I had an idea this was going to be an interesting session.

6

OPERATING IN
A BURNING BARN

COLONEL DALE WAS ESPECIALLY WELL KNOWN FOR HIS FAMOUS hunting stables. He also trained the First City Troop, the ultra-fashionable cavalry corps who appear in their original 1776 uniforms at official gatherings in Philadelphia. I had heard a good deal about the colonel's estate and it certainly came up to expectations. There were eight barns, some old, some new, plus a carriage house containing a lordly Park drag, a landau, a graceful char-à-banc, and a Stanhope phaeton. Later I found out that each of these vehicles was kept in perfect condition and had its own team or teams of carriage horses. I remember especially an exquisite little spring house with green shutters under a tremendous sycamore and a hollow oak so huge that a children's playhouse was easily set inside. I drove past fields of yellowing corn, around a pond so big it was almost a lake. There was an island in the center where a pair of Canada geese lived. I drove by fields where cattle and horses grazed, past little clapboard cottages, the homes of the estate employees. At last I arrived at the stables.

The colonel was waiting for me. He was an impressive figure, 6 feet 4, with snow-white hair, and he turned out to have a formidable British accent. He led the way to a box stall some 20 feet square that held the biggest stallion I'd ever seen. I filled two stainless-steel buckets with warm water and added a little disinfectant. When I was ready, Colonel Dale called over two grooms.

"Get a chain shank on him," he ordered.

The men knew their business but for a while I thought the stud was going to win. He fought like a wild animal, throwing the grooms against the sides of the stalls. When they finally got the shank over his nose and were able to restrain him, the colonel turned to me.

"Do you think you'll be able to do the washing up?" he asked doubtfully.

"I don't intend to try without tranquilizing him first," I said.

The colonel said no one had been able to inject him for years. He watched while I got out a hypodermic syringe with a special small, sharp needle. While I filled it, Colonel Dale said bluntly, "The instant he feels the prick of that needle, he'll go berserk and the men won't be able to hold him. I hope you know what you're doing."

One of the things I'd learned from Dr. Charles was how to give an injection. He was an expert as it was so often needed with temperamental racehorses. When the syringe was ready, I walked over slowly to the stallion while the grooms hung onto his head and he struck out with his hoofs, showing the whites of his eyes. I talked and stroked him until he had quieted down a little. I had scrubbed my index finger well and I gradually pressed the finger against a nerve in the neck so as to deaden it. Then I slipped the smallest gauge needle in under my finger. He never felt it. I squeezed in 1 cc., then 2 cc., still not daring to breathe. I could feel him beginning to relax. I pulled the needle out and thank heaven it didn't break. They sometimes do, no matter how careful you are. After a few minutes' wait, I was able to wash him up without trouble. When I left, Colonel Dale said, "My regular veterinarian could never have done that. I'm afraid he's getting too old for the work. Would you be willing to take his place?"

Sometimes it is a nice moral question whether you are justified in superseding another veterinarian. Ethical standards are extremely strict on this issue. This was the only time I ever came close to infringing the rigid code. Even though I needed the job desperately, I wouldn't have taken it without at least speaking to the former veterinarian if it had not been for a freak case that occurred a few weeks later.

Although the colonel had told me that I was to become his

regular doctor, his former veterinarian still came to the stables. Colonel Dale didn't have the heart to tell him that he was no longer needed and I was glad he did not. It would have broken the old man's heart. The colonel was boarding a Canadian mare and foal at the time. The mare had foaled in Canada and her owner wanted her rebred immediately. When a mare has given birth, she typically comes into "foal heat" on the ninth to the twelfth day after and can be bred at this period. Personally, I think this is taking too great a risk. The mare is usually in too weakened a condition to be successfully bred so soon. However, this mare's owner had shipped her and her newborn foal, which, of course, was nursing and had to be with her dam, to the Dale stables because the colonel had this famous stallion. As it turned out, the foal had not been able to endure the long trip and had developed pneumonia. So instead of getting two foals, the Canadian ran an excellent chance of not getting any—his first one dying of pneumonia and the mare not settling after the hurried second breeding.

Colonel Dale's old veterinarian had examined the foal and told him that the case was hopeless. So the colonel sent for me, obviously as a last chance. Young as I was, I knew that strictly speaking I should have refused to see another veterinarian's patient, but I happened to know that this doctor had made a number of disparaging remarks about "this female so-called veterinarian," and I couldn't resist the temptation to see what I could do.

When I arrived at the Dale stables, the filly foal was lying on her side, breathing heavily. She had a temperature of 104 degrees and I was inclined to agree with my rival: the case was hopeless. Still, there were new drugs and new techniques I was sure the old man had not employed. I decided to try my best.

The foal was badly dehydrated and had no reserve of strength. She had been too weak to nurse from her mother for several days and was half-starved. I began by getting fluids into her veins and a new antibiotic. When she looked a little stronger, I gave her an injection of B-12, at that time one of the new "miracle drugs" that were just coming in. I worked over her for three hours, and at the end of that time I saw her stagger to her feet and begin nursing from her mother. It was one of the proudest moments of my life.

When I returned the next morning, the foal's fever had broken and she was doing splendidly. Colonel Dale was delighted but worried that his old doctor would return and find me there. "If he does come, please take off your coveralls and hide your bag. Then I can say you're only a visitor," he begged. I didn't like this idea at all but the colonel added, "I wouldn't want to hurt the old man." That was different and I agreed. Colonel Dale kept his word about taking me on as his regular veterinarian, although he still had the old man make occasional calls. Only once did he come while I was there and I barely had time to hide my bag and change my clothes. Luckily the old gentleman soon retired, which was just as well as I went at least once a day to the Dale stables for the next twenty years.

In spite of all my difficulties, it was wonderful to get away from books and studies and be with live animals again. I was never a "booky" person, and I hated the long periods of study and theory rather than practice. I also enjoyed driving through the lovely countryside so rich with history. Near the Pennsylvania Railroad tracks between Malvern and Frazer is an isolated little graveyard I often passed. In 1832, there was a cholera epidemic here that struck down a number of Irish laborers who were putting the line through. The only doctor was the local blacksmith, who claimed to have some knowledge of herbs. As the Irishmen were Catholics, some nuns came out from Philadelphia by stagecoach to nurse them. Despite their efforts and the blacksmith's good intentions, fifty-seven of the immigrants died and were buried in a hastily improvised little graveyard surrounded by a low stone wall built by their friends. Unable to find a stage to take them back to the city, the nuns returned on foot. Because they were Catholics, no one would take them in, give them food, or even a drink of water. It is hard to believe there was such prejudice and cruelty only a little more than a hundred years ago. I think of it every time I pass the forgotten little graveyard.

Most memories are more pleasant: old St. Peter's Church, built in 1744 and originally a log cabin; the eight-sided schoolhouse at the corner of Diamond Rock and Yellow Spring roads, built in 1818 by the German and Welsh settlers; driving along the Brandywine, and Crum Creek. The arbor vitae hedges, the vast tulip poplars, going to the various stables (often old dairy barns redone), talking to farmers who remembered bringing in all their supplies by ox cart from the Trenton Cutoff Railroad. It was still hard to convince people that a woman could be a veterinarian, especially a "horse doctor," but slowly I was becoming accepted. People began sending for me not only because no man was available but because they had confidence in me. Sometimes, partly by luck, I could pull a really startling diagnosis. Once I was called by the distracted owner of a breeding stable to hear that his mares were all aborting, no one knew why. He had had several veterinarians in but none of them could find the cause. I was clearly the last hope.

I've always had a good nose and even as I walked into the stable, I could smell mold. I sniffed around and found moldy straw in the stalls. Although the mangers were full of prime hay, the mares were eating some of their bedding, enough to cause them to abort. That man became a walking advertisement for Dr. Lose. "She didn't even have to make blood tests or examine the mares," he would assure a group of impressed listeners. "Just took one look around and told me what was wrong." I wish I could do that more often.

I was too busy looking after other people's animals to have any pets of my own, but at this time I adopted—or to be more accurate, was adopted by—one of the nicest animals I've ever known. Although I like all animals, there is one species that doesn't seem to like me. For some reason, cats go out of their way to bug me. I try to be nice to cats. I call them "pretty pussy," scratch them under their chins, and sometimes slip them a shot of milk. It does no good. The moment I appear, one cat says to another: "OK, pal, here's Phyllis Lose. Let's drive her nuts." If I lay down a clean white towel and turn my back, when I return there are little dirty black footprints all over it. If I put down a tuna fish sandwich, it's inside the nearest cat before I can retrieve it. Cats are innately curious. They love to see what I've hidden in the bottom of my bag, even if that means throwing everything else out; they do scarf dances with bandages; they play pitty-pat

119

with my freshly sterilized instruments. In short, if cats ever turned out to be an endangered species, I could choke back my tears.

Then I met Nancy. Mother first noticed her while I was examining horses at a famous racing stable. Mother suddenly said, "That cat belongs to you, Phyllis." I looked around and there was a kitten, tiger-striped, sitting up watching me. She was unlike any other cat I'd ever seen, not only in her appearance but in her actions. When I scratched her head, she accepted my advances gravely, then followed me around the stables, watching everything I did, sitting up on her hind legs like a dog begging, something I've never seen a cat do before or since.

Always a veterinarian, I gave Nancy (I forget how we knew her name was Nancy) a physical examination and then treated her for parasites, a treatment she badly needed. Most cats would have resented this, but Nancy took it in such good part that when I got ready to leave, she jumped onto the seat of my car, curled herself up, and started purring. When I tried to get her to leave, she was insulted. At last I went to the owner of the stables and asked if I could buy Nancy. "Take her," he assured me. "Frankly, I think she's a witch's familiar. She gives everyone the creeps." So we drove home with Nancy sitting beside me and Mother saying proudly, "I told you she was your cat."

Nancy made a quick check of the house, selected the kitchen as her headquarters, and moved in with us. Whenever I went on my rounds, Nancy would accompany me. She always followed me around, checking on me carefully and sitting up in her funny, doglike manner so she could see better. She lived with me for many years and I will never have another cat. None could come up to Nancy.

As my practice began to expand, I needed an assistant. I had plenty of offers but soon discovered that finding a good assistant is a very difficult job. Just being willing is not enough. The assistant must be willing to learn, must be able to think fast in an emergency, must have a good memory, must have courage, and must possess a certain amount of physical strength. Last of all, and perhaps the most important, your assistant must be tireless— as you must be. You must both be ready to keep going for forty-eight hours without rest, driving long distances in the worst of weathers, and often walking considerable distances if the sick animal is out in a pasture. After a long time, I got a girl named Barbara Miller to help me. She was from Scotland and had worked with British veterinarians. She was very capable and fearless with animals.

I should explain here that as a young girl, I had hunted three days a week with the Radnor Foxhounds. One of my heroines in the hunt was Mrs. Jean DuPont. Mrs. DuPont was a daring though not a reckless rider; a lady who believed in formality, she always rode sidesaddle and was followed by two hunt servants impeccably dressed in "browns" with tweed caps. At that time—in the late 1940s—many people were followed by their grooms, who opened gates for them and also were there in case of spills, which in the Radnor country were fairly frequent and could be dangerous. You never see this any more but in those days it was taken for granted.

I was fifteen then and had no grooms to follow me, so I stood in great awe of Mrs. DuPont. I knew her stables were internationally famous. She had a magnificent place near Newtown Square, then the center of the horse country. She was especially well known for her Welsh ponies. She had them imported from all over the world, selecting only the best for conformation, ability, and disposition. She had well over a hundred, and what I would suppose to be one of the finest collections of carriages to be found anywhere. The carriages were and are kept in the loft of one of her great barns. I was once allowed to see them; each is kept in perfect condition, the brasswork shined, the leather oiled, and the woodwork painted and varnished. Mrs. DuPont often hitches up a team of her ponies to one of the carriages and drives around the estate. She is a regular exhibitor in the carriage class at the Devon Horse Show, where every sort of horse-drawn wheeled vehicle is shown, from farmer's hay carts to elegant phaetons, gigs, landaus, char-à-bancs, lordly Park drags, and tallyhos. Mrs. DuPont also has several sleighs, equipped with bells, that she drives in winter when there is snow on the ground. To me, she represented everything that was knowledgeable and elegant in the horse world.

Although I was too impressed by the great lady ever to approach her, I think Mrs. DuPont must have been conscious of my adoration as a child, for she always went out of her way to speak to me in the field and remembered my name. One day in particular made a great impression on me. The hounds had lost and then found again. As they struck the line, they broke into full cry and went streaming off, the master after them sounding "Gone away" on his horn. One always follows the master—it is a basic rule of fox hunting—but Mrs. DuPont, after studying the lay of the land and thinking for a minute or so, deliberately turned her horse's head and rode off in another direction, her grooms following her. After a moment's hesitation, I followed her. This was the only time I'd ever ignored the master, but I was certain that Mrs. DuPont must be right.

It was a terrible run: fences, ditches, hedges, and woods. Mrs. DuPont on her big hunter took every obstacle easily but I had a harder time on my little mare. Finally, Mrs. DuPont drew rein. We were on a little hill and below us the fox was running, the hounds way behind him. In some way, she had known exactly what he would do. The pack had left the field far behind and we were the only riders in sight. The fox went to ground in a few minutes and we had the honor of being the first up. I was most impressed. Mrs. DuPont had shown that she could think like a fox, which isn't easy to do.

Although after I had gotten my veterinary license and had a few years' experience I was fairly confident of my abilities, I never dreamed of being called on to treat any of the DuPont horses. Only the top veterinarians could expect that. Then one Sunday morning, the telephone rang. I sighed and answered it. Barbara resignedly got up and began checking items.

It was a man's voice on the line. "I'm the foreman at the DuPont stables," he informed me. "We have a bad case—a big thoroughbred colt that was castrated yesterday morning and is hemorrhaging badly. I doubt if anyone can save him but please come at once."

"What about your own veterinarian—the man who did the castration?" I asked. After my experience with Colonel Dale's old veterinarian, I had sworn to be scrupulously careful about ethics.

"He went away for the weekend right after the castration and his wife can't refer us to anyone. Please hurry. The colt is pretty near dead."

"I'm on my way," I said.

The DuPont estate was very familiar—I knew my way from hacking through. We turned in a big gateway and drove up a mile-long drive bordered by sugar maples. We passed by a lake where a flock of Canada geese were floating, then acres of pastures, each enclosed by trim white fences. At last we came to the stables, which were kept cleaner than most houses. The foreman was waiting impatiently and took us at once to the stall where the poor colt lay.

He was a big chestnut, in a cold sweat, his anxious eyes bloodshot. There were five grooms with him trying to keep him calm but he was then walking in constant circles, mechanically as though on a treadmill. He was clearly out of control with pain. A stream of blood as thick as a lead pencil squirted from his genital region and the stall looked like a slaughterhouse.

I am always optimistic when dealing with a sick animal. I take for granted that my patient is going to live. This was one of the few times I felt despair.

"Get me a bucket of warm water—quick," I told one of the grooms, while Barbara raced back to the car to get the necessary instruments. I gave him a sedative and a coagulant to control the bleeding, but I saw I would have to get in as quickly as possible and ligate the open vessel. I did not dare do it until I had washed my hands and was surgically clean; otherwise I would be almost certain to infect the wound.

I washed my hands as quickly as I could while waiting for the sedative to take effect. It was terrible to stand there helpless watching this splendid animal bleed to death but there was nothing I could do until I was clean and he stopped walking. The men could not hold him; they'd already found that out. At last, I was able to apply the hemostats to the open cord. It was the remains of the cord and the tunica vaginalis (the inside of the scrotum) that were hemorrhaging. A horse can withdraw these tissues up into his body; if he had done so, there was virtually no way I could reach them to apply the hemostats. I moved slowly, talking to him quietly, gradually raising the hemostats toward him. Finally he stood still, his head hanging, and I was able to clamp them on. Instantly the blood stopped, as suddenly as water stops flowing from a spigot when the handle is turned. For the first time, I began to have some hope.

With catgut ligation, I sutured the open vessel. Then I gave him a brief examination. His mucous membranes were almost white, he had lost so much blood.

"Get the I.V.'s with replacement fluids," I told Barbara.

"I already have," she said.

While the intravenous fluid was running into the tortured animal's veins, I removed the remains of the large membrane with a scalpel. Afterwards, I took several yards of gauze and pleated it into the wound, holding it in place with a few sutures. Then I gave my patient an injection of antibiotics. I looked at his gums again: they were turning pink. The watching grooms knew what that meant and cheered.

"Check him every hour to make sure the bleeding doesn't start again," I advised. "And keep him very quiet. Don't even lead any other horses past him. I'll be back in a few hours."

A natural question is why Mrs. DuPont's regular veterinarian, who was a most capable and experienced man, had made such a mistake. He had performed what is generally considered to be a routine operation, then left for his holiday without bothering to check if there were any side effects or whether this particular animal had responded to the gelding differently from most. In nine cases out of ten, this would have been safe enough; but in all medical work you must allow for the individual and for the unexpected. I've always tried to remember that.

When Barbara and I came back the next day, Dean the foreman was there to greet us. The colt was doing well, better than I'd dared to expect. After giving him another injection, Barbara and I were preparing to leave when the foreman said, "Mrs. DuPont would like you to take over her stables as her regular veterinarian. No, wait a minute!" as he saw I was going to object. "It isn't only because of this. She has been planning to change veterinarians for some time." Then he told me that the other veterinarian was suffering from certain emotional problems that made it difficult for him to practice. In fact, I had already heard about it. Gratefully, I took the position.

What I've always regarded as my most terrifying experience occurred at the DuPonts'. I certainly hope never to go through such a nightmare again.

Mrs. DuPont had had a mare shipped in from California. She was in foal and the trip had been too much for her. The foal had begun to come but the mare was unable to deliver it, so Barbara and I were called in. It was evening when we started out, the sky already darkening, the wind beginning to rise, and I knew a thunderstorm was on the way. It looked like a bad one.

The foreman rushed us to the stable as the storm clouds towered over the maples. Two grooms were standing beside the mare, who was down on the floor. "We tried to keep her up, Doctor, but it was no use," the foreman explained. The head and neck of the foal were protruding from the mare's pelvic canal, and it took only the briefest inspection to show that the baby was dead and had been dead for some time. In fact, tissue change had set in and the little corpse was cold. I carefully evaluated its position and found the dead foal firmly wedged within the mother's body. The shoulders were against the pelvic rim and the legs were doubled back. When the head and neck of a foal are out, it is a serious business. They have to be repelled into the mare's body so you can get hold of the forelegs, straighten them, and start pulling. Under these circumstances, saving the mare would be difficult.

"Shall I get the 'unmentionable'?" asked Barbara. The "unmentionable" was a box that contained instruments I used only in cases of extreme dystocias, that is, difficult births. Such instruments are used only in cases of last resort, and they look more like devices employed by medieval inquisitors than modern doctors. I realize it is unscientific and even childish but Barbara and I never liked to admit even to ourselves that the box existed. Hence the nickname. A fetotomy must be performed.

"Yes, and several I.V. bottles," I told her. While she was gone, I gave the mare an antibiotic injection and a sedative and took her temperature. It was 105 degrees—very high.

The mare had her eyes rolled back and was so exhausted from the struggle that she could scarcely move. I told the grooms to fill my stainless-steel buckets with hot water and then opened the "unmentionable" box Barbara had carried in. From it, I took out a wire saw, chains, a collection of special knives, and a hook. Meanwhile, Barbara had slid a needle into the mare's vein and was pouring in the first of the I.V. injections.

Outside, the wind was growing increasingly stronger and flashes of lightning made every detail of the stall stand out as though etched in fine golden wires. The rumble of the thunder was coming closer and louder. The mare's uterus was so dry I had to inject mineral oil to lubricate the dead foal and then push the corpse back into the mother. I tried to find the forelegs but they were doubled so far back that I could not reach them. Finally, I had to put both arms into the mare, holding a braided wire that cuts like a saw when worked back and forth. To protect the mare's uterus, the wire had to be threaded through a pipe except where it came into contact with the foal. Once it was in place, I screwed handles onto the wire's ends. I would have to cup up the dead foal in the mother's body and remove it piece by piece. It was a grisly affair but there was no other way.

Now the storm broke, such a storm as I have never seen before or since. The lightning seemed to be in the room with us and the concussion of the thunderclaps was stunning. I am not afraid of thunder and lightning but this was like being in the center of the storm itself. I had to wait between claps to shout instructions to Barbara, who was trying to help me. The electricity crackled around us. You could smell the ozone. The flashes were so brilliant that the stall lit up with an uncanny brightness as though giant yellow searchlights were being rapidly switched on and off within yards of where we were working. Each flash would be instantly followed by the paralyzing crack of the thunder like a hundred cannons firing in unison; then would come the long rolls whose reverberations shook the building.

Under ordinary circumstances I would have taken refuge in a cellar or some other protected spot, not from panic but from normal common sense. However, we could not leave the mare. The I.V.'s had to keep going into her and I had to free the foal. Part of the body came away, allowing me a little more room in which to maneuver. I got the chain and worked it over the foal's pastern. Some veterinarians use a rope for this purpose but a chain does not slip as a rope does and holds traction better.

I was still trying to get the chain into position when there came another flash, even closer and more dazzling than the others, and the crash of thunder that followed it left me dazed. Suddenly all the lights went out.

"Get a flashlight!" I shouted to Barbara, both my arms still deep within the mare and numb from pressure and reduced circulation.

"I don't dare stop with the I.V.," she called back.

"You'll have to hand it to one of the grooms. Run for the car!"

She dashed out of the barn while I continued to work by sense of touch. Then I saw through the stall window what seemed to be an aftermath of the flash. There was an ocher glow that instead of fading grew steadily stronger. At first I thought there was something wrong with my eyes; the intense glare of the lightning had caused a persistence of image. But the light grew more intense and I could smell smoke. The barn must have been struck by lightning.

I saw the beam of the flashlight jerking about like a luminous rod as Barbara ran with it down the passageway. The barn was full of horses. We would have to abandon the mare and try to get them out.

"The barn next to this one has been hit," gasped Barbara. "The whole thing is in flames. I can hear cattle mooing inside."

"Leave the flashlight and see if you can help them," I told her, still trying to get the chain in place.

Barbara ran out. Now I could hear the sounds of the terrified animals as well as the crackle of the flames. There was little need for the flashlight as the fire lit up the stall. At last the chain slipped into position and I tried gently to pull out the remains of the foal. I could not move it. Then I got the hook, slid it into the mare's body, and pulled with that. Nowadays, I would not attempt a fetotomy of this nature. I would have the mare taken to my hospital and there perform a Caesarean. A Caesarean is a difficult and somewhat dangerous operation, but nothing compared to this sort of thing. Even if the foal's body is finally successfully removed, the shock to the mare will often prove fatal or damage her reproductive tract irreparably.

At last there was nothing for it but to take my knives and cut away the fetus, bit by bit. It was sickening, bloody work. The floor was covered with blood when the remains of the foal finally came clear. Just as they did so, a man came in with a flashlight. He took one look and shouted, "Oh, my God!" I thought he was going to faint.

"Don't worry, I saved the mare," I told him. "Help me get her on her feet."

As we got her up, Barbara returned. "There are men at the barn but I don't know if they got the cattle out or not. The heat's so strong I can't get close to it," she panted.

"Start giving the mare some more I.V.'s and I'll take a look," I said, although what I could do I had no idea. I ran out into the rain. It was coming down in a solid wall that formed sheets where the wind struck it. The drops were the size of marbles and hit the ground so hard that they rebounded. The walkway between the barns had become a stream that poured over my boots. I saw a little group of men coming around from behind the barn, silhouetted against the flames. I ran toward them.

"Did you get the cattle out?" I shouted over the tempest.

"They broke out themselves," one of the men called back. "That's hay and straw that's burning now. Several tons of it."

It was a disaster, but at least no animals had been killed. I returned to the horse barn, and Barbara and I worked on the mare until we were sure that she was out of danger. That was five hours from the time we first arrived. I'm happy to say she staged a complete recovery and later had several healthy foals.

7

I JOIN THE CIRCUS

For several years, I had been friends with a big, blond, blue-eyed girl named Audrey Bostwick. I had known her ever since veterinary school. Our class had been taken to see her parents' stable in Chestnut Hill, just outside Philadelphia, called The Monastery. The stable had stalls for twenty or twenty-five horses and was rightly considered a model of its kind. Audrey's mother had always been very fond of horses and kept a number of hunters and fine driving horses. Audrey shared her mother's interest. When our class arrived, Audrey walked up to me and said cheerfully, "Hi, you probably don't remember me but I've seen you ride in the shows." Right away we were talking horses while the rest of the class inspected the stables.

After that, Audrey and I became good friends. Her family had always been greatly interested in the Philadelphia Mounted Police Department and through Audrey I got to know several of the mounted policemen, especially an Inspector Charles Turner who was always particularly nice to me. When the growth of the city finally engulfed The Monastery, the Bostwicks sold it to the police, who used the stable for their horses. After I had become a veterinarian, I occasionally dropped in at The Monastery and Inspector Turner would sometimes ask my advice about the chargers—police horses are always referred to as "chargers" in memory of the days of cavalry. He knew that although I specialized in horses, I was interested in all kinds of animals and was willing to tackle anything from a vulture with frozen feet to a boa constrictor who had burned his belly crawling over a hot radiator. I think this impressed him, as many veterinarians won't touch the so-called exotic animals, partly because there's always a danger in working with them (that vulture bit off part of my ear) and partly because they don't know how to treat them. I didn't either; I just did my best.

A few days after attending the mare at the DuPonts', I got a call from Audrey. "What do you know about polar bears?" she asked.

"Absolutely nothing," I assured her, "except that they are big and mean and I hope never to have anything to do with one."

"That's too bad because Ringling Brothers and Barnum & Bailey are in town and they have a sick polar bear. Something wrong with one of its paws. They called the police department to ask if there was a veterinarian who would handle dangerous animals and Inspector Turner recommended you. He called me as he didn't have your number and I said you'd be right over. The circus is at the Spectrum and you're to ask for Ursula Bottcher. She's got the bear act. Goodbye and good luck."

I packed up my equipment and started for the Spectrum, feeling most unhappy.

Ringling Brothers and Barnum & Bailey claimed to be "the biggest show on earth." Actually it was twice that big. In fact, it had become so gigantic that it split into two shows: the Blue and the Red. One show plays in the East and the other in the West. These shows rotate on alternating years. Neither goes under canvas any more. There are several reasons for this, the main one being the difficulty of finding lots near cities large enough to hold the gigantic Big Top. Both shows travel by train (no more romantic colored wagons drawn by teams of huge dray horses). They usually spend at least a week in any one location.

In Philadelphia, the circus generally plays in the Spectrum, one of the city's largest arenas, in south Philly. The show unloads on the Food Fair distribution center, which has a separate siding large enough to accommodate the tons of apparatus, and the performers are transported by buses to the Spectrum. The animals go by truck, except for the ones that can be easily handled such as the elephants and the horses. They have to walk. There are some 200 performers with the circus plus about 150 workingmen (propmen, riggers, grooms, roustabouts, etc.), and over 200 animals, so transportation is quite a problem. However, the circus is so well organized that in the days before World War I, the German general staff sent over a group of officers to travel with it for a few weeks to study the techniques of moving great numbers of men and animals (in those days horses and horse-drawn vehicles were the only form of military transportation) easily and quickly across country.

The circus had its own veterinarian, the famous Dr. J. Y. Henderson, who divided his time between the Red and Blue units as well as paying occasional visits to the menagerie in Venice, Florida. As Dr. Henderson was no longer young, this constant traveling naturally put quite a strain on him; nor could he be in three places at the same time. This was why I had been called in.

I found a spot in the vast parking area surrounding the Spectrum and hurried over with Barbara to the arena. I was expected, and one of the grooms (all the men who take care of animals are called grooms) took us through the lines of cages to where the polar bears were kept. There I met Ursula Bottcher, who had been waiting impatiently for us. She was the last person I would have expected to be a wild animal trainer. She was small, only a little over 5 feet, blond, and looked delicate. Behind her in their cages were the bears, ten of them, moving back and forth with the peculiar swaying manner of bears. I could see that several were limping.

"When did they start having trouble with their feet?" I asked.

Now we had our first problem. Ursula, it turned out, was German and spoke no English. I had forgotten what German I had learned in college. Ursula's husband was also there, a quiet, retiring German who also spoke no English. There seemed to be no one to translate. This was a poser. While I was trying to recall some of my German, a very pretty young woman came up in a costume composed mainly of feathers. She wore a blue cape with

131

a red lining and had the biggest eyes I have ever seen. She had obviously just come from the ring and was on her way to her dressing room.

"You are no German speaking?" this apparition asked. "I am German. You are the doctor, no? You tell me what you want to say and I make it into German. My name is Jeanette Williams."

Jeanette, it turned out, was one of the big stars, and exhibited a troupe of Lipizzan stallions from Vienna. We were to become great friends. She chatted with the worried Ursula and then translated in her odd but just comprehensible English.

"Polar bears are making very delicate and can't have sawdust sprayed with any petroleum product," she informed me at length. "Often this is done to make away with the dust. Always we try never to use such sawdust but sometimes a mistake makes itself and we get the wrong kind. Then the bears get like an eczema on their paws. Look once!" She pointed to the bears' feet and I could see big red sores.

I moved closer to the cage to get a better look, but Ursula grabbed me and pulled me away.

"What's the matter? Their paws are too wide to go through the bars," I pointed out.

Ursula spoke rapidly and Jeanette explained, "They are making clever enough with their paws to turn them sideways and slip them through. Then they are after hooking their claws in your clothes and pulling you against the bars where they can get at you. That is not good."

I was sure it wasn't. But if I couldn't get close to the bears, how could I treat them?

This, of course, is a major problem in treating nearly all wild animals. I did not know it then, but I was looking at what most trainers consider the most dangerous and unpredictable of all creatures, including the big cats. The polar bear is the second-largest land carnivore in the world, surpassed only by the giant brown bear of Alaska. Unlike other bears, which live largely on vegetables, the polar bear is a hunter who eats virtually nothing else but flesh. A big male may weigh up to 1,600 pounds and be 9 feet long, standing 5 feet at the shoulder.

It seemed to me that the best treatment for the sores would be a cortisone antibiotic preparation. The question was how to apply it.

"Suppose I put the medicine on some cotton, tie the cotton to the end of a long stick, and rub it on that way?" I suggested.

Ursula shook her head violently when this idea was translated. "She says no," explained Jeanette. "The bears are grabbing the stick and eating off the cotton."

I had a sudden inspiration. I went out and bought an aerosol can containing a cortisone preparation. Then, from a safe distance, I sprayed the bears' sores. I came back the next day and the next to repeat the treatment. Within a week, the bears had recovered.

No matter how busy she was, Jeanette always took time off to act as my translator when it concerned animals. This devotion to animals turned out to be typical of nearly all the circus people I met. Elvin, Jeanette's husband, went out of his way to help anyone who seemed to be in trouble. Elvin was a "flyer," a trapeze artist, and one of the best in the world. He was an Englishman, always beautifully dressed, and one of the handsomest men I have ever seen. He was a world-famous aerialist and noted as a daredevil.

With Jeanette as translator, I learned quite a lot about bears. They are especially difficult to train because their expression does not change and you never know what they are going to do next. Another problem is that once angered, nothing stops them. They are indifferent to guns fired in their face, to water shot from powerful hoses, even to fire. If you try to hold a bear off with a chair as you can a lion, the bear will probably take the chair away from you and beat you over the head with it. Not even the best trainers can always handle them. Jack Bonevita, who taught Clyde Beatty, was killed by a polar bear. On the other hand, polar bears are quick to learn—when they want to. They have even been trained to carry lighted torches. Being hunters, they have better vision than other bears. They also have longer necks, which they can extend to a surprising distance; "snaky" is the only word I can think of to describe them. And they have surprising memories. William T. Hornaday, for many years the director of the New York Zoological Park in the Bronx, tells of a big male polar bear who was captured by boats while he was swimming from one ice floe to another. Because of that, he never went swimming again, even on the hottest days.

Ursula's arms and sides were covered with scars but she was absolutely fearless in working the bears. In her act, she actually danced with one bear twice her size. I heard a number of stories about her. Once during winter quarters while rehearsing her troupe, one of the bears tore loose a section of the cage and ran into the stands where a number of the circus hands were watching. A man who witnessed the escape told me, "I never saw people scatter so fast, not even when a lion or tiger got loose." Ursula didn't hesitate a moment. While her husband kept the rest of the bears in the cage, Ursula grabbed a manure shovel, ran into the stands, and beat the bear over the head until he returned to the cage. He could easily have killed her. She just had him bluffed.

Ursula told me that she had a hard time keeping the bears white. Their fur had a tendency to turn green. It was mainly a question of diet. They had to have certain kinds of fish and certain sorts of bread. The cages had to be kept scrupulously clean. Polar bears' feet are heavily haired to protect against the cold and to make it easier for them to hold onto ice, and this seems to be one reason why the right sort of sawdust is so important, as most kinds get under the hair and produce an irritation.

Although everyone was very nice to me, I had a certain feeling that they were being rather formally polite, as though I were an outsider who wasn't really to be trusted. But after Ursula's bears recovered, people went out of their way to say hello and do me small favors. Neither Barbara nor I ever had to carry a thing; there were always half a dozen people ready to do it for us. I treated a few other animals, mainly horses, and then I was asked to treat an elephant.

Elephants have always fascinated me although I had never met one personally. The show had sixteen elephants and their biggest "bull" had gotten a bad laceration on her leg (in the circus, all elephants are called bulls although actually they are all females). Most circus elephants nowadays are Indian elephants, which are far more tractable than African. The African elephants are bigger, have much larger ears, and considerably heavier ivory, and at one time it was considered a matter of pride for all circuses to have at least one African elephant. Barnum's famous Jumbo, probably the largest elephant ever to be exhibited, stood 10 feet 10 inches at the shoulder and weighed several tons. He was surprisingly gentle and children could ride on his back. Poor Jumbo was killed by a locomotive one night while crossing some railroad tracks. He was probably the greatest animal attraction in history.

Another German couple worked the elephants—for some reason, many of the wild animal acts had German trainers. The trainer was Axel Gautier, and he had a helper named Shad, a big woman, very dark-skinned, in striking contrast to her Nordic employer. I had seen them working with the big animals on my previous trips to the circus and was much impressed by the care they took of their huge charges. In hot weather they hosed them down immediately after they had appeared in the show, not even taking time off first to change their own elaborate costumes.

Now Axel led me over to my patient, who was chained to stakes by one front and one hind leg. He spoke to her in German, and the "bull" reached out with her trunk and felt my coveralls with the tip. An elephant's trunk is surely one of the most curious, sensitive, and complex structures in the animal world. It has tremendous power. A blow from it can easily kill a human being or even a lion. Yet the tip is so delicate and sensitive that an elephant can pick up a blade of grass with it. I afterwards found out that the clasps that hold the chain around the elephants' legs have to be specially constructed so a man needs both hands to release them; otherwise the elephants could open them with the tips of their trunks. Elephants can also turn on faucets whenever they want a drink. To date, no elephant has ever learned to turn one off again, though.

The cut would have to be sutured, which would obviously hurt the elephant. Then she would have to have an antibiotic injection. I was quite sure she wouldn't like that either. Ordinary catgut sutures wouldn't be strong enough to close the laceration in her thick hide and I had no idea how much antibiotic to use on an elephant.

"Her name is Bertha," Axel informed me, patting her trunk. Bertha swung her trunk back and forth and looked at me unpleasantly from her little pig eyes. It was clear that if she didn't like having needles stuck in her, there was nothing in the world Axel could do to prevent her murdering me. At this moment, I heard a curious swishing noise behind me, like a number of fans being waved. Nervously, I spun around. Only a few feet from me a line of elephants was marching past, each one holding the tail of the one in front with her trunk. Their vast padded feet made absolutely no noise; the swishing sound came from their waving ears. At the end of the line was a baby elephant not much bigger than a pony. The baby refused to grab the tail of the elephant in front of her and this made the groom angry. All elephant grooms carry sticks 3 or 4 feet long: at the end is a hook perhaps 2 inches long. These hooks are the only means the men have of controlling their giant charges. If an elephant misbehaves, the trainer catches the hook in some tender part of her anatomy, usually where a leg joins the body, and jerks. It's hard to believe that the hooks can really produce any impression on an elephant, but they do. To discipline the baby, the groom gave him a nudge with the hook. Without looking around, the little elephant kicked backwards and sideways. His foot caught the man in the belly. He doubled up like a jackknife and went flying over a heap of props. Slowly he rose and limped away, still doubled up.

"Can all elephants kick like that?" I asked Axel. The laceration was on Bertha's right foreleg, a perfect place from which to launch a kick, and Bertha was a lot bigger than the baby.

"Yes, they are good kickers. I think they can do more harm with their feet than with their trunks, although I am not being sure."

I took a deep breath.

"Mr. Gautier, I am not an elephant veterinarian."

"I am knowing."

"I really work only with horses."

"I am knowing."

"I have no idea how to suture that cut or what dosage to give Bertha."

"I am knowing."

"Also, to tell you the truth, I'm scared to death of her."

"That I am also knowing. You want to start now? Shad and I

will stand by her trunk. Perhaps with our hooks we can keep her from hitting you with it; perhaps not. I am hoping you can duck quick. For the kicking, there is nothing we can do."

Well, if he was willing to take a chance on me, I'd take a chance on him. The laceration was showing signs of infection and was covered with flies. I considered.

Barbara spoke up. "We have some stainless-steel suture material in the unit with some larger surgical needles. How about using them?"

"Good idea. And get my biggest syringe; the one that holds thirty cc. I know the correct dosage for a horse and I'll just have to figure out how much more Bertha weighs than a horse."

When I had all my instruments laid out, Axel and Shad moved in on either side of Bertha's head. I took a deep breath, bent over, started cleaning the cut, and instilled an anesthetic. Once the local block took effect, I sighed with relief.

Bertha swung her trunk around and I expected to be knocked halfway across the tent, but Axel stopped her with a little gentle pressure from his hook. After that, she stood like a stuffed animal while I sewed up the 3-inch cut. Then I lifted my syringe filled with antibiotics and stood puzzled. I could see no place in the thick hide to insert the needle.

Axel saw my problem and with his hook pointed to a place between the right foreleg and the body where the skin was thinner. I gave the injection and got out of the way as fast as I could, although there was no need for me to worry. Bertha was better disciplined and steadier than most horses. There was one other difficulty, the flies. They were still settling on the laceration by the score. Luckily, I'd foreseen this and was prepared for it. I had left large loops, which we call "rabbits' ears," on the sutures. Barbara got me a big sterile gauze sponge out of our car and with the rabbits' ears I tied it securely over the cut.

After that, I was called in several times to treat one of the elephant herd for minor matters. They are surprisingly delicate and need constant attention. Their feet have to be treated for sores, calluses, and cracks; they must be brushed and their skins oiled. Their diet is important and must be carefully watched. Not infrequently they fight among themselves, and separating two enraged elephants isn't easy. They seem to take strong likes and dislikes to certain people. If they dislike you, it is well to keep out of their way.

Except for the great apes, I believe that elephants are the most intelligent of all animals and I know they can remember and execute at least two dozen commands. In the old days, they helped put up and take down the tent, and I have been told that in India the working elephants seem to take pride in their jobs and show amazing skill in handling the big teak logs, knowing exactly what angle to send them down the chutes into the river and the easiest way to haul them.

Bertha made a complete recovery. As a reward, Axel asked me if I would like to ride her around the lot. I know it's foolish, but I was as delighted as a child. On command, she held up one leg. I mounted on that, grabbed the harness on her forehead, and with her trunk she boosted me onto her back. Not until I was actually on top of her, straddling her neck while holding onto her harness with both hands, did I realize how truly big an elephant is. It looked a mile to the ground and her head was the size of a picnic table. When she moved, it was with a curious, lurching, twisting gait that I can't describe except that it twisted every bone in my body. Learning how to be a mahout must take a lot of practice. Once around the lot was enough for me.

But my most difficult circus patient was a young leopard. Jeanette and Elvin were raising it for her brother, who had a cat act. One of his leopards had had kittens. She had rejected them, which animals that are constantly kept on public display often do, and as the man didn't have time to raise them himself, he asked Jeanette and Elvin to help. All the kittens had died except one and this one had developed a bad cold. She was about one-third grown and weighed around 60 pounds.

"She is making not good," Jeanette explained, as we went to the Williamses' really magnificent trailer. "She is tame—for a leopard. She does not bite as hard now as she will later."

When we entered the trailer, I noticed that the Williamses were careful to shut the door after them. This meant the leopard was loose in the trailer, something I hadn't expected. They had to look around for her, and at last found the cat lying sprawled out on their bed. Elvin scratched her under the chin and she purred happily. Then she jumped off the bed and came toward me, snarling. I have said that I don't get along with cats for some reason. Just because this one was spotted and ten times the size of an ordinary cat made no difference. She walked around me snarling and spitting. All I could see was teeth. Then she rubbed against my leg. "See, she likes you!" said Elvin happily, but I wasn't deceived. The leopard was only trying to see what kind of a rubbing post I'd make before sharpening her claws on my leg.

I decided to give her an injection of penicillin, although cats respond so differently to drugs from other animals that I was nervous about it. I filled my syringe while the leopard continued to pace around me. I could imagine what she'd do when I stuck a needle into her.

"Ready!" I said nervously. Jeanette and Elvin diverted her attention and I shoved the needle in. The leopard let out a scream like a banshee and leaped a foot before spinning around, but I had shot in the dose and gotten back. I also wanted to give her nutrical to build up her strength, but even when we concealed it in chicken, her favorite food, she refused to eat.

Then I had an inspiration. "Smear it on her paws," I suggested. "Cats hate to have anything on their paws. Maybe she'll lick it off."

We tried it and the leopard retired to the bed, angrily licking her paws. I felt that I'd won.

Unfortunately, that was only the first round. A couple of days later, I had to give her another shot. This time pussy knew what was coming and also was much stronger—she had been eating a little since my first visit. All she needed was to see the needle to go crazy with rage. Jeanette and Elvin had to put on heavy cowhide gloves with gauntlets to hold her down. The third time was even worse. They couldn't control her and had to call in a young lion trainer named Jewell New. The three of them were able to hold her, but just as I pulled out the needle, she twisted around and struck out with one of her long front legs. Her claws raked New's arm, leaving three nasty gashes. He assured me he was used to being clawed by cats, but that was the last time I treated the leopard. Cats' claw marks nearly always infect because they are covered with decaying food. As the claws are retractable, the film of rotten meat stays on them and does not wear off while the cat walks about as it does on a dog's claws.

I saw quite a bit of Jewell New after that. He was a tall young man, just starting out as a lion trainer, completely dedicated to his career. He told me there was one lion that hated him, he had no idea why, and he could never turn his back on that animal. No matter what other lion he was putting through his paces, he had to keep one eye on this particular cat. "And then there's Buddy," he added. "I'll show you Buddy."

Buddy was in a cage by himself. New went in and Buddy leaped on him. For an instant I was shocked, but it was immediately apparent that the 400-pound cat was playing. New rolled around the floor with Buddy like a man wrestling with a big dog. Later, New gave me an exhibition of Buddy sitting behind him with his paws on the man's shoulders while New drove a motorcycle around the ring. "Buddy taught himself that trick," New explained proudly. "Once while I was on the motorcycle, he ran over and jumped up behind me. I think he's the only motorcycle-riding lion in history."

It seems to me that people are either fascinated by cats or instinctively dislike them. Except for my dear Nancy, who was more like a dog, I have always been a little nervous with them. Other people react in just the opposite way. I was told that in 1962, a young novice from the Convent of the Good Shepherd in London took some children to a circus. After seeing the lion act, she left the convent and joined the circus as a lion trainer. The legendary Mabel Stark, who was probably the greatest tiger trainer in history, as a girl of seventeen went to see the old Al G. Barnes Show and a trainer asked if she'd like to go with some of his tigers, thinking the girl would be terrified at the idea. Mabel walked in, and when a Sumatra tiger glided toward her with that terribly suggestive crouching movement only a cat can make, the girl walked over to him as though going to meet a sweetheart. The startled tiger hesitated, then turned and jumped back to his pedestal. I think I can honestly say that I've never been afraid of a horse no matter how mean he was, but the big cats do frighten me.

Everyone I talked to who worked with the big cats had a

couple of set phrases they always repeated. "Cats can be trained but they're never tame," and "The last words of every lion trainer are, 'That's the one cat I thought I could trust.'" New admitted that even Buddy might turn on him for some inexplicable feline reason. It sometimes seemed to me that cat people are so obsessed with their fierce charges that they talk of nothing else (which, of course, isn't really true). They speak a special language as they sit around the grease-joint (the wagon that serves circus people their meals), drinking coffee and talking of their experiences.

"Last month in Syracuse, I had 'em pyramided [the cats sitting on pedestals of various heights with the boss cat on top] and called out Sheba, my Barbary lioness, for the roll-over [cat lies down and rolls over on cue]. Pete—he's a big Bengal [tiger]— hates her guts. I saw him getting ready for a heavy jump [coming down heavily to kill instead of springing down lightly just to get off the pedestal]. You know how a cat's pupils get big and his tail stiffens when he means business? I flicked him with the whip so he'd come at me instead of Sheba. He came, all right, and mauled me bad. I had to blank him in the mouth [fire a blank cartridge]. Every show since then he'll try to get me when I cue Sheba. Right after she's finished, I can play with him like a dog. I don't, though. People think he's a killer so they keep coming back, hoping to see him get me."

I must admit I can't see the charm of working with animals that occasionally not only kill but eat their trainers. I suppose the fascination stems from their great physical beauty and also from their self-sufficiency and eternal resentment of any kind of discipline. A man armed with only a chair and a whip has no more chance in a cage with the big cats than a baby among werewolves. His real weapon is understanding cat psychology so perfectly that he outguesses them. This constant outguessing is so difficult that trainers plan on spending at least one-fourth of their wages on hospital bills. No life-insurance company in the world will issue them a policy.

Most cats used in show business are newly caught wild animals; the cage-raised kind have learned too much about man's weaknesses. An adult cat costs about $5,000, and the trainer may invest a whole year's profits, saved by skimping on his own and his family's comforts, to buy a new animal that he probably must order sight unseen. The first glimpse of his purchase is a tense experience because trainers believe they can tell a cat's nature by such signs as the set of his eyes, width of forehead, reaction to noises, and interest in food and people. The trainer studies the new arrival more anxiously than he would a child he is considering adopting, for the man intends to trust his life to the animal's instincts.

Cats charge in two ways: a "business" charge and a "bluffing" charge. A real business charge is almost impossible to stop. In a bluffing charge, the cat is simply annoyed and trying to drive the man away.

The trainer begins by sitting near the cage for hours until the foaming animal stops trying to get at him. Then he starts feeding the prisoner. Sooner or later the cat comes to tolerate him. When the man decides he won't meet a business charge, he quietly enters the cage.

He must go in alone, for the cat is his baby. No one else can know enough about that particular animal to help him intelligently. His gun is loaded with blanks, for no bullet is apt to stop a cat in time and also the man will risk a great deal to avoid killing a valuable cat. He can't wear armor because he has to move quickly and he can't even carry a spear because the prick would drive the animal wild. So he carries nothing but a kitchen chair, a blunt pole, and the impotent gun.

The cat may not come at him immediately, but eventually he will. If it's a business charge, that's it. But if it's a bluffing charge, the man can divert it with his pole. It's a cat characteristic that they'll usually stop and bite at any object thrust toward them. The cat bites the pole, probably thinking it's part of the man, and hurts his mouth. But sooner or later he'll knock the pole aside and come in snarling. The man stops him with the chair. The animal is puzzled by the four legs poking at him simultaneously; he doesn't know which one to attack. At last he gets bewildered by this five-armed wooden creature and retreats. This is the crucial part of the whole training: when a cat first admits defeat.

No one can predict exactly what a cat will do then. Some spring over the chair and the trainer must quickly shorten the pole and rap the animal on its sensitive nose. Others get panicky.

I saw a young lioness dash around the arena, ricochet off the sides, and nearly land on top of the trainer. The man finally had to stand in the middle of the cage, well away from the sides, until she quieted down. Some cats never give up but will fight the pole and chair indefinitely. These animals are usually sold to zoos.

When the cat stops charging, he is "seat-broken." A big block seat is used, or four pedestals put together, and the cat is teased with the pole until he jumps onto it. Then he is left alone to quiet down. Gradually, three of the pedestals are removed, until the cat recognizes his own seat and leaps to it as soon as he enters the arena. Then the trainer calls, "Up high!" and the cat is taught his place on the pyramid seats at the back of the cage. Seat-breaking and pyramiding are the bases for all acts.

Generally, a trainer doesn't have too much trouble with cats until he tries putting them together. They usually neither like nor dislike their trainer, but lions have a very strong feeling about each other. There's always a boss lion that rules the arena and there's always some ambitious young male who is trying to displace him. The trainer has to make sure the old fellow is never put at a disadvantage or the younger male will kill him. Then often two lions get "pally" even in the few minutes each day that they meet in the big cage; if the trainer punishes one, the cat's friend will go for him. And if there is a female in heat, every male in the arena goes frantic and the trainer may get killed trying to keep them apart. He can't drop the lioness out of the act because in circus work the whole routine is timed to the second and she has to do her part. Here a veterinarian might be some help by administering drugs to keep her out of heat for a period.

Tigers seldom show any interest in one another. If a pair gets into a fight, the others rarely interfere; but in a lion tangle, every lion in the arena jumps down to help his friends. Mixing lions and tigers is extremely dangerous. The two are natural enemies although they are so much alike physically that they can inter-breed and produce a hybrid called a *tiglon*. Trainers who put on mixed acts often count on losing two or three animals every season.

New told me, "People ask me if we train the cats by kindness. That's like asking if a sheep can train a hungry wolf by kindness. Many men who know something about animals think we train them as you would big dogs. Cats don't think like dogs. I've never seen anyone succeed in house-breaking a lion or tiger or teaching one to retrieve, which is simple with dogs. Cats aren't stupid. They just have no desire to please you and they don't connect punishment or reward with a trick as a dog does."

While seat-breaking a cat, the trainer watches for a certain characteristic of the animal that suggests a trick he might do. Some lionesses have a nervous habit of whirling around like a dog chasing its tail. If a trainer sees one do this, he encourages her until she'll do it on cue. When he signals her to start spinning, the band strikes up a waltz, making sure to keep time with the cat. The audience thinks the lioness has been trained to dance to music.

All cats have certain traits that can be developed into tricks. Most of them dislike jumping down from a high place. In the wild, they catch their prey by running it down after a stalk, not by dropping on it from above. This characteristic makes possible the well-known barrel-walking trick. The trainer puts a big barrel beside the pedestal, chocked so it can't roll. The cat is teased with a pole until he jumps onto the barrel. When this becomes routine, the cage boys fasten ropes to the barrel and roll it slightly. The cat rapidly shifts footing, like a lumberjack on a log, to keep from having to jump. This same action makes the barrel move even more but the men control it with their ropes. Finally the cat will leap to the barrel and roll it across the arena by his fast footwork.

Cats can't be trained to do anything against their natural impulses. All the standard arena tricks—pyramid, teeter-totter, lie-down, hoop jumping, walking on blocks, sit-up, and barrel walking—depend on some phase of their psychology. For many years trainers thought that no cat could be taught to roll over (a simple trick for a dog) because there was no way the cat could be induced to perform the action until it became routine. Finally, a smart trainer noticed that some of his charges would reach up to play with the lash of his whip, just as a kitten will lie on its back and bat at a waving finger. He got a lion to lie on his side and strike at the lash. Then he moved the whip very slowly across his body, the lion rolling over to follow the dangling tip. When the routine had become established, he omitted the whip and the lion rolled over when he waved his arm. A new cat trick had been created and is now a standard feature.

The secret of all "lion taming" is to establish a certain habit-pattern in the cat's mind. Although cats are the most individualistic of all animals, once they get into a specific routine, they seldom break it. If a cat is used to jumping to a pedestal placed in a certain spot, he'll refuse to jump if the pedestal is moved 2 feet away. Trainers sometimes deliberately misplace a pedestal so they can put on a show of cracking whips and shooting off guns, none of which affects the cat in the slightest. Finally, the man quietly kicks the pedestal into place and the cat instantly jumps to it. The crowd goes wild.

The "door-rusher" is a perfect example of absolute dependency on routine. Often when a trainer turns to leave the cage, some cat will charge him. Instead of trying to break the habit, the man teases the cat, encouraging him. The habit-pattern becomes established and the cat charges automatically, hurling against the bars as the man slams the gate. The audience thinks the trainer has barely escaped with his life. Occasionally substitute trainers, not knowing about the door-rusher, have been killed; but ordinarily the cats are so completely ruled by habit that they'll turn and trot back to their pedestals even though they may have knocked the man down on their charge.

This automatic response to routine has saved several trainers' lives. One trainer told me, "Once I had to give a show after a heavy rain and the floor of the arena was covered with straw to give the cats a better footing. I was trying to make a young tigress take her seat when I slipped and fell. Sheik, a big Bengal, grabbed me by the thigh. His teeth sliced through the flesh and then I could feel them grate on the bone. I knew my leg must be nearly severed, but my cage boy rattled the chute door. That's the signal for the cats to leave the arena. Sheik promptly dropped me and ran for the exit. Then he remembered me and turned back. By that time I was on my feet again and could handle him."

Jeanette also had a "cat" act. She had two magnificent cheetahs, the "hunting leopards" which for hundreds of years were trained by Indian rajahs to run down game like greyhounds. They are the fastest four-legged animals in the world and although true cats, they are doglike in many ways. They have nonretractable claws like dogs and can be tamed—and I mean tamed, not just "trained." Jeanette, who was wonderful with horses, had trained a Morgan to allow the cheetahs to ride on his back and afterwards, together with a cheerful little mongrel dog Jeanette had found wandering around the lot, they rode in a cart pulled by the Morgan around the ring. Jeanette had no trouble with the cheetahs; the trouble was in finding a horse that would put up with the two big cats, each weighing about 100 pounds. It was a very pretty act, and seeing the three species of animals, all natural enemies, working together and obviously enjoying it, delighted the crowd.

One afternoon I got an emergency call from Jeanette. She was usually a very level-headed person but this time she was so mad with rage I could scarcely understand her. All I could gather was that something had gone wrong—very wrong—with the Morgan and I was to come at once.

One trouble with circus work was that it cut into the time I was able to devote to my regular patients and routine rounds to the farms. This always worried me. There were times when I regretted that I'd ever agreed to help out at the Big Top, much as I enjoyed it and found it a wonderful change from my usual practice. However, this time there was no doubt that something was seriously wrong and I dropped everything to race to the Spectrum.

When I arrived, Jeanette was still so furious she could only express herself in German, so I had to talk to Elvin.

"You know our groom," he began. I remembered the man well. He was little, tough, hardworking, and deeply interested in horses. His great fault, from what I could see, was that he overestimated his knowledge and occasionally took it upon himself to do things without consulting Jeanette. Usually he was right in what he did, but with animals one bad mistake can ruin your charge. Still, he was so conscientious and reliable that Jeanette kept him on. But now Elvin told me: "The Morgan threw a shoe. Instead of getting the blacksmith, our groom tried to put on a new shoe himself. The shoe was too small and he tried to rasp the hoof down to fit it. As a result, the horse has gone dead lame. We have two shows a day to give and if Jeanette can't go on, there'll be an empty ring."

It sounded bad. "Let me see him," I said.

I took one look at the hoof and was almost as mad as Jeanette. Mistakes happen, everyone in the horse world knows that, but a stupid, pointless mistake like this that could have easily been avoided is criminal. The pulsation in the foot was bad, and it was hot. The whole hoof was badly mutilated.

I gave the poor fellow a sedative and an anti-inflammatory injection. Then I packed the hoof with cotton soaked in iodine. This was the trick good old Willy Bradley had shown me when I was a little girl. Afterwards, I got some black tape and taped the packing in place. I used black tape so it would match his other hoofs and not be noticeable, as I was still hopeful that he could go on for the afternoon show.

It was ten minutes to show time. The Morgan was walking normally. Luckily, he didn't have to perform any stunts; just trot around the ring pulling the cart with the cheetahs and the dog. Jeanette walked him once more, slowly, around the lot. Suddenly she gave a cry. He had gone lame again.

I ran to him. By the greatest of bad luck, he had stepped on a sharp pebble. I pulled it out but he still limped. I looked at Jeanette's and Elvin's anxious faces. I knew something they hadn't told me; with the circus it's "No show, no pay." The horse would have to go on if it were even remotely possible.

I did something I have never done before or since: I gave him an injection of lidocaine in the foot. This desensitizes the nerves for a time so the horse feels no pain. In the show ring or the racetrack it is illegal although sometimes done. Jeanette's music was starting. Doubtfully, she began to lead the Morgan toward the ring. He moved perfectly.

"Get the cheetahs!" she called to Elvin, while she and I hitched the Morgan to the cart. She made her entrance a little late, but the clowns covered for her with some pranks, and started around. I stood watching, not daring to believe the Morgan would make it. The act went over without a hitch, drew its customary applause, and I was able to breathe again.

The next morning, the hoof was only slightly sore. I re-packed

147

it and the Morgan was able to go on in the afternoon show without an anesthetic. I kept changing the packing for the next two days. A week later, I showed the circus blacksmith how to put on a wide web-bar shoe, with all inner surfaces concaved out. From then on the Morgan was perfectly sound, but his other shoes had to be adjusted from week to week to mask his bad hoof as it grew back into shape.

Jeanette's main act was a "liberty act" in which she used ten Lipizzan stallions. These are the "stallions of Vienna," famous for their dressage or "high school" feats. The horses perform a capriole (leap up with front and back legs extended), the courbette (rearing up with folded front legs and hopping forward on hind legs), pirouette (keeping back legs still while spinning in a circle), and many more amazing feats. In a liberty act, the horses are not ridden. They circle the ring while the trainer stands in the middle and directs them by voice and a long whip. On command, they change direction, break up into groups of two or four, rear together, come toward the trainer, and perform other feats like an equine ballet. It is my favorite act.

I had heard so much about how graceful Lipizzans are that I was somewhat surprised the first time I saw them. They are chunky, about 16 or 17 hands at the shoulder, and resemble a Morgan. They are one of the oldest breeds. Originally they came from Iberia in Spain. (Even though they have been in Austria since 1564, their stable is still referred to as the Spanish Riding School.) Three times they have had to be evacuated from Vienna to keep them from being captured by an invading force: once at the time of Napoleon, once during World War I, and again during the last war to save them from the Russians. Colonel Podhajsky, the director of the school, took the horses to an estate some 200 miles from Vienna and appealed to General George Patton to protect them. Patton was an old-time cavalryman who loved horses; he gave them sanctuary until the Russians left. (Walt Disney made a picture about the rescue called *The Miracle of the White Stallions*.)

Curiously, all Lipizzans are born black and only turn white between the ages of four and ten. They have two sets of movements, called "on the ground" and "above the ground," the latter when the horses spring into the air as in the capriole. I thought that I knew something about horses but until I saw Jeanette exhibit those Lipizzans I had no idea what horses can do under a really skillful trainer. All my life I have regarded stallions as being temperamental and potentially dangerous. I never heard of two stallions being left alone together; they would be certain to kill each other. Yet Jeanette kept her ten stallions tethered side by side along a rope. I would not have believed it possible.

I became professionally involved with the Lipizzans when Pacco, her lead horse, went lame. Pacco was the most important horse in the act. He always entered the ring first, the others trailing him, and set the pace for the rest. He was the only stallion that could perform the amazing capriole. At one point in the act all the horses stopped, spun around, and then continued going. During this maneuver, one of the other stallions stepped on Pacco's hoof and injured his coronary band.

Pacco was a big horse, 16 hands 2 inches, and weighed about 1,800 pounds. When I went over to examine him, I asked the heartbroken Jeanette which leg had been injured. She spoke to Pacco in German and he instantly raised the hurt leg and held it out so I could check it. I have often thought that horses are quite as intelligent as dogs and could be taught virtually everything a dog can do, but few people ever take that much trouble with them. My examination also showed that Pacco was having trouble with his hocks and stifles, the joints in the hind leg, as he was getting old. He would need an operation, and it would take several weeks for him to recuperate.

As the show was going into winter quarters, Jeanette decided to have the operation performed in Florida. A few days later I got a call from Jeanette. On the way to Florida, while Pacco was being transferred from a van to a boxcar, his leg had been caught between the train and the ramp. This time it was hopeless. Pacco would never perform again.

Yet for Pacco, at least, the story had a happy ending. He was retired as a stud to a breeding farm where there were a number of mares. Pacco, I imagine, was far more content there than doing caprioles for even the most appreciative audiences.

8

CIRCUS HORSES

I ENJOYED BEING WITH THE CIRCUS PEOPLE. THEY WERE UN-like anyone else I had ever known. Those I knew seemed to have no interests outside the circus and were totally absorbed with their act. Their act represented everything to them: their livelihood, their pride, their social position, their skill. For this reason, they seldom mixed with "townies," as they called everyone not with the show. Although invariably everybody had been nice to me from the moment I first walked on the lot, it was not until I had treated several animals that they really accepted me as a person, no longer a "townie." Even though the circus is constantly on the move, it always remains the same. It is a separate world, maintaining its own code, its own language, and its own privacy, no matter where it is. Many of the performers are foreigners, often speaking little or no English. Most of the time I doubt if they had any idea where they were, nor did they care. They were part of the circus and what went on outside the sawdust rings did not interest them.

I had had the idea that circus people were generally tough, often unscrupulous gypsies, who were ready to take advantage of innocent "rubes" in any way they could. After talking and being with them, I came to the conclusion that circus people are one of the most exploited groups in the country. Because they are constantly moving, communities take advantage of them. They have no friends away from the lot. They are in no position to bargain, to make demands, to stand up for their rights. They have no chance to do any comparison shopping, and if they are over-charged or sold shoddy goods, they have no recourse as they must move on and can't appear in court. Even in my case, al-though the lives of very valuable animals depended on my skill, they had no way of knowing if I were a good veterinarian or a bad one. They just had to trust Inspector Turner's recommenda-tion.

However, though I liked them and I think that they liked me, I got two of the worst shocks in my career with the circus.

For the last three years, whenever Barnum & Bailey's plays Philadelphia, I have been called in to provide veterinary service. One year I was asked to castrate an enormous Belgian stallion who was in the rosinback (bareback) act. He was so big seven people could stand on his back at one time. The act is called the rosinback because the horse's back is sprinkled with rosin so the performers have a firmer footing. The stallion was invaluable, but unfortunately he had grown so aggressive that he could not be trusted. It was decided to geld him. His owner was a Bul-garian who spoke only a little English and whose whole life was apparently wrapped up in this giant animal. The stallion was, I think, the only thing in the world he owned except the clothes on his back; he was also his one source of income. He had put off having the stallion gelded as long as possible until it became obvious that it was either that or having him put down.

As the stallion was both big and old, it would be a far more difficult operation than with a young colt, so I decided to take the stud to the Philadelphia Mounted Police Stable where I would have some privacy and sturdy-built stalls. With their usual kindness, the police were willing to let me use their facilities. But there was a problem: the horse was too big to fit into their horse ambulance. That meant he would have to be walked to the hos-pital, in Franklin D. Roosevelt Park, nearly a mile from the lot along city streets crowded with traffic. The police generously assigned me a squad car to go ahead of the horse and instructed traffic officers to stop the cars at the various intersections we would pass. I decided to make the trip late at night when the traffic would be at a minimum.

We started off well enough, the squad car at the front with its flashing light revolving, followed by the Bulgarian leading the enormous Belgian, with me in my veterinarian car bringing up the rear. Everything would have been fine except that the Bulgarian insisted on leading the horse down the center of the street. That, of course, halted traffic both ways. I stopped my car, jumped out, and tried to explain to him that he should keep the horse as close to the curb as possible. Either he wouldn't or couldn't understand. Before we had gone more than a few blocks, traffic began to pile up on all sides. Then the police tried to get the man to pull the horse over, but he stubbornly continued to stick to the middle of the street. When we finally got to the stable, it seemed to me that half the motorists in Philadelphia were cursing us.

My niece Margaret and my sister Norma set up instruments and assisted me. I performed the operation which, as I had foreseen, was a long and difficult one. Standing castrations on an adult animal always are. In addition, it was late at night—or rather, early in the morning—I had been working all day and was tired. The strain of the long walk amid honking horns and shouting motorists hadn't been easy, either. To top off everything, the horse's owner insisted on standing beside me during the operation, breathing down my neck and giving me instructions in Bulgarian that I couldn't understand and really didn't need. By the time it was finished, I was crying tired. Then the animal had to be gotten back to the lot and tied to the picket line. I checked him just before I left. He was in excellent shape and I felt proud of the job I'd done.

Once outside of Philadelphia, I stopped at a diner for a cup of coffee as I was so tired and dizzy that I didn't trust myself to drive. While I was sipping the coffee, I heard the car radio in my car (parked just outside the door) buzz and squawk, then our code for an emergency. "What now?" I thought, and gulped the rest of the coffee before running out. Whatever it was, someone else would have to handle it. I was done in.

Mother was on the radio. "Phyllis, get back to the circus as fast as you can," she told me. "That horse you gelded is hemorrhaging badly. There's blood everywhere and the owner doesn't think he can live."

"That's impossible!" I gasped. "He was doing perfectly when I left."

"He isn't now. Something went wrong. You'd better hurry."

I started the car and raced back to Philadelphia. I was almost as sorry for the Bulgarian as for the horse. But what could have gone wrong? All the way to the lot I kept trying to think of some mistake I could have made, but the operation had seemed faultless. It is very seldom I ignore traffic regulations or exceed the speed limit; I certainly did both this time. Even so, it was almost a certainty that the horse would be either dead or dying before I could get there.

I tore onto the lot, killed the engine, and, grabbing my bag, ran for the section where the horses were kept. There was the Bulgarian, waiting for me. He beckoned me wildly and started running for the picket line. I panted after him. Thank heaven, the Belgian stallion was still on his feet at least. What was more, he appeared to be quite all right. Puzzled, I followed his owner, who anxiously bent over and pointed to a tiny spot of blood near my suture.

"He is making blood!" shouted the man, in an agony of apprehension.

I don't know which I felt more strongly, relief or anger. A wound must drip a little, otherwise it would infect. I tried to explain this to the man, but he kept repeating "Blood! Blood!" over and over again. At last I was able to find another Bulgarian groom who could speak enough English to understand the situation. Even so, when I left, the horse's owner was standing watching the minute spot of blood with all the anxiety of a devoted mother. I was so exhausted by my long day—I had been over twenty-four hours without rest—and the nervous tension of thinking I had killed the horse through some mistake that I seriously considered lying down on the asphalt lot and going to sleep. But the circus was beginning to wake into life, it would be impossible to sleep, and besides I was sure the worried Bulgarian would be after me every few minutes with some fresh report about his horse. So I decided to go back to our farm, driving slowly and forcing myself to stay alert until I was able to stagger up the stairs and collapse on my bed.

The other bad shock I had at the circus was nobody's fault

except mine. Some newly arrived horses had developed shipping fever and I was called in to treat them. Shipping fever generally is the result of a change in diet and water plus general weakening from long confinement. I arrived at the lot in the evening and as I got out of my car, I noticed a gang of teenagers who were wandering around the outskirts of the lot obviously up to no good. I got out my bag and took the precaution of locking my car carefully before going to the horse lines.

I had no trouble telling which were the sick animals. They stood hanging their heads, with a mucous discharge from their nostrils. They were running temperatures of from 104 to 105 degrees. None was in really serious condition and I had some colic medicine in the car which I'd found was virtually a specific for this trouble. I returned to the car, got the medicine, relocked it, then remembered that I'd noticed some lacerations on a couple of the horses, so I unlocked the car again and got some cauterizing powder. Then I went back to treat my patients.

I was putting my instruments away when I realized that I had forgotten to lock the car after getting the powder. This may not seem too serious to you but it could have come close to ending my career as a veterinarian. My car was full of narcotics of various kinds and I had to give a strict accounting every month as to exactly how many drugs I had used and for what purpose. In fact, the laws are so strict that I could never throw away a syringe for fear it might be found by a drug addict. For once I had come away without any assistant so I had no one to help me.

I remembered the youngsters snooping around the lot. They could clean out the car in a few minutes and I could never give a satisfactory explanation to the Federal Narcotics Bureau. Sick with apprehension, I ran out. As I approached the car, I saw the worst had happened. I knew I had left the door closed. Now it was open and bottles and instruments lay strewn on the asphalt.

First, I checked the narcotics. Wonder of wonders, none were missing; nor were any of the instruments gone. Only one item had been stolen. Years ago, Mother had given me a rather handsome purse which I always carried with me. Usually I kept small sums of money in it, credit cards, keys, and so on, but of late I had put all such items in other places. I still kept the purse on the dashboard, more as a good luck symbol or a keepsake than anything else. Now the purse was gone. The kids had not realized that the drugs and some of the instruments were worth a small fortune and had thrown them aside looking for money. For sentimental reasons, I would have liked to get the purse back, and I advertised in the papers for it, knowing the youngsters had undoubtedly thrown it away after finding it empty. No one answered my ads, but even though I was sorry to lose the purse, I was so relieved they hadn't taken any drugs I could think of nothing else.

In my ordinary work with horses on the Maine Line, there were several breeds I seldom got to see. This was one of the great appeals the circus had for me. There were the Lipizzans, big Percherons for the rosinback act, thoroughbreds for a spectacular race around the tent, hunters for jumping exhibitions, bridlewise saddle horses for the Garland Entry (an intricate quadrille on horseback in which the performers trot in and out of great hoops covered with flowers), and western stock horses for the Wild West Show. The circus is one of the few places where horses are encouraged to exhibit their smartness. One trainer told me, "When you're training a horse for show purposes, you spend five minutes training him and two hours trying to figure out what's going on inside his head."

I was particularly struck with the rosinbacks. I had always taken for granted that all a rosinback had to do was canter around the ring while the performers did tricks on his back. Actually, I believe it's harder to train a good rosinback than it is most trick horses. The horse must canter at exactly sixteen beats to the complete circle and his tempo can never vary. You can only find about one horse in twenty who will do it correctly.

When a rosinback first starts out in the ring, he gets dizzy from going around in a circle and the trainer has to give him frequent rests. But finally the horse is able to keep going for hours without a break. Timing is all-important. If a girl leaps into the air from the back of a moving horse, does a split, and then comes down again, she must be absolutely sure that the horse will continue to canter at precisely the same speed. If the horse moves slightly

155

faster when he feels the girl leave his back, she will come down on his slippery rump and suffer a bad fall. Often a performer who falls will crash into the ring curb and this generally means a few broken ribs, if not a broken neck.

A trainer told me that when he was starting out, he used conventional word signals with his horses, including the traditional "Whoa!" when he wanted them to stop. As the climax of his act, he had five girls run across the ring together and all jump simultaneously onto the horse's back. During one show, the girls were in the act of jumping when a man in the audience suddenly shouted, "Whoa!" The well-trained horse instantly stopped and the girls went over his back. Fortunately, they missed the ring curb so none of them was seriously hurt. "Just the same, I'd have killed that man if I could have told who it was," the trainer told me vehemently.

After that experience, he trained all his rosinbacks to stop on another command instead of "Whoa!" He wouldn't tell me what the command word was.

One of the best trainers of circus trick horses in the country is Mark Smith, a chunky little man who crossed the southwestern deserts of California in 1912 with his family in two horse-drawn wagons and has been working with horses ever since. Mark was called in by producer Sol Lesser, who was making a film entitled *Peck's Bad Boy at the Circus*. The script called for a child bareback rider to do a back somersault from one rosinback to another with both horses going at a canter around the ring. There were several adult performers who could do this dangerous feat but no child had ever attempted it. The regular Hollywood horse trainers told Lesser that it was impossible. Then Lesser heard about Mark Smith and went to him.

"I knew at once that everything would depend on the horses," Mark explained. "Any child trained in acrobatic dancing could make the back flip, supposing that the child had nerve enough to do it on a horse's back. But the horses would have to be absolutely steady and the rear horse would have to stay exactly in position so he would be perfectly placed when the child came down."

Mark got a ten-year-old girl named Gwendolyn Gillespie from

a school of dancing. Gwen was a plucky kid and very cool-headed. The big problem was finding the horses. Mark had one rosinback named Buddy he could trust, but he needed two. There was only one other rosinback Mark had ever seen to which he was willing to trust a child's life, a gelding named Runt whom Mark had trained while he was with Al G. Barnes Show. When Mark telephoned the circus he was told that Runt had long ago been sent off to auction with a bunch of other circus horses past their prime.

Mark, helped by his brother Pete, spent a wild week trying to find out what had happened to Runt. The old Percheron had been passed from one dealer to another. At last, Mark found that he had been sold to a dealer in northern California. Hitching up a horse van to their car, Mark and his brother raced to the town, praying that Runt was still there.

When they arrived at the dealer's, they found the man in the act of selling the Percheron as a cart horse. The old circus trooper was standing there abjectly while the two men bargained over him. "Poor old Runt was the most miserable-looking horse I've ever seen," Mark explained. "He had two shoes off, he hadn't been curried for weeks, and he was covered with bites. The dealer had penned him up with a bunch of tough mules and they'd torn him up plenty."

When Runt saw Mark, he began to whinny frantically and tried to run to him. The dealer turned on the two Smiths and demanded, "What the hell's going on here? This sale is closed. Keep away from that horse." The Smiths are inclined to be a bit hasty at times and Pete knocked the dealer sprawling. When the man got up, he was in a more reasonable mood. Mark paid him off. Then he and Pete led the Percheron into the trailer while the astonished farmer stood goggling at them.

Mark gave the rosinback a few days' rest in his stable. Then he led the horse into the practice ring. When Runt saw the familiar ring, he pulled out of Mark's hands, jumped the ring curb, and stood there pawing the sawdust, waiting for the signal to begin.

In three days, Gwen Gillespie was able to do the back flip on the horses' backs. After the scene had been shot, Mark pensioned Runt off on a big ranch where the old horse could spend the rest

157

of his days quietly wandering over the hills with other retired veterans.

One of the handsomest and most intelligent of all horse breeds is the Arab. I was once called on to treat a horse at the Russian Circus when it played Philadelphia. I must admit that I was a little apprehensive about the Russians. I thought of them as being people who would show little desire to cooperate with a capitalistic veterinarian—and a woman at that. I certainly got a surprise when I arrived on the lot. Such clicking of heels, outstretched hands, and friendly eagerness I had never seen. All their horses seemed to be Polish-bred Arabian stallions, magnificent animals in perfect health. But the trainer took me away to a quiet corner where there was a small spotted pony at the far end of the stable area suffering from rhinitis, an inflammation of the mucous membrane. I don't know what she did in the show but she was obviously the trainer's special pet and he worried over her as the Bulgarian had over his Belgian stallion. The poor little animal was quite ill and I decided she had better spend some time in the hospital. When this was explained to her owner, he was most downcast and asked if he could stay with her. "I will gladly sleep in the stall with her if there is no room for me," he assured me. I told him that wouldn't be possible and he watched sadly as she was loaded into the horse ambulance and driven away. He called twice a day to know how she was doing and on his free day came out to stay with her. Fortunately, the pony made a good recovery or I am sure her owner would never have forgiven me—or the United States. As it was, I think we made a friend of him.

While at the Russian Circus, I had a chance to examine the Arabs. These noble animals are the oldest domesticated breed of horses in the world, and in the opinion of many horse lovers, the finest. They remind me of our American quarter horse, which was developed from the mustang and has Arab blood. The quarter horse was originally trained as a stock horse in the West, herding cattle. He had to be able to run at a good clip for a quarter of a mile—hence the name—which was all that was necessary to overtake a wayward steer. Unlike a thoroughbred, he was not required to run at great speed for considerable distances, nor did he need to know how to jump; instead, he had to be able to perform a number of equine feats connected with herding stock. A good stock horse must be able to canter in a tight figure 8, changing leads—that is, changing the foot with which he takes his forward stride—as he passes through the center of the 8. He must be able to spin (whirl around on his hind legs), pivot (make a turn of 180 degrees), back, and break instantly from a walk to a canter. In addition, when his rider ropes a calf, the horse must immediately slide to a figure 11 stop (slide on his hind legs so that they make two parallel marks on the ground). He must then keep the rope taut while the rider, after hog-tying the calf, crawls back and forth under the lasso to show that the horse is steady.

A really good stock horse can work a herd of cattle as a sheepdog does a flock of sheep. Without a rider, he can canter into the herd and cut out any animal indicated by his master, keeping it away from the others and holding it in position to be roped. Exhibitions featuring stock horses are growing increasingly popular, but unfortunately, in my opinion, the horses are being bred down in size so that they can turn more quickly and perform even more remarkable feats. I am sure this is a mistake. As the horses grow smaller, so do their heads, and they become less intelligent and less muscular. To compensate for these drawbacks, the training is often done cruelly with viciously sharp spurs. All this is self-defeating, as are all over-adaptations. But I would like to see an Arab trained as a stock horse; I have the feeling they would be very good.

The training of "trick" horses, usually for the motion pictures, is an art in itself. The horses have to bow, wrinkle up their lips as though laughing, nod and shake their heads for "yes" and "no," and play dead by lying down on their sides. Teaching a horse to perform tricks is very different from training a stock horse. The routine performed by a stock horse is based on a horse's natural abilities. A wild stallion will habitually lead a herd of mares; he also knows instinctively how to change leads, pivot on his hind legs, and slide to a dead stop. The trainer's job is to teach the horse to perform these feats at certain definite times and in a certain way. When a stock horse goes stale after taking part in too many ring exhibitions where no cattle are used, the trainer puts the horse on a range for a few weeks and lets him work with real cattle. There the horse learns that these various stunts he has been taught have a definite use. He can then be brought back to the show ring and will perform with fresh interest.

There is no way of encouraging a trick horse to take an interest in learning tricks. A horse can't see any reason why he should pick up a handkerchief on cue and bring it to his trainer or walk over to a lady and put his head in her lap. Dogs can be taught tricks fairly easily because dogs have a natural desire to please their masters. But horses are far more independent. The only way to teach a horse tricks is to put him in a situation he dislikes and can avoid solely by some action that can later be developed into a trick.

A horse is generally taught a trick in four stages. If he is to be trained to kneel, the trainer begins by lifting one of the animal's forefeet. Horses find it difficult to stand on three legs so the horse comes down on his knee; finally, the horse learns to kneel quickly and easily as soon as the trainer lifts the foot. This is the first step. The next comes when the horse learns that it is easier for him to kneel immediately when the trainer simply touches the foot, rather than to have the man pull his leg off the ground. The horse is now said to "kneel on cue," the cue being the trainer's act of putting out his hand and touching the knee. Later, the horse learns to kneel when the trainer merely extends his hand toward the foot. After that, the trainer can stand a dozen yards away, raise his hand, and the horse will promptly kneel.

This form of training is simply an extension of the method by which a saddle horse is taught to answer to the reins. At first, a horse turns left or right only because his rider pulls the bit in that direction and the horse moves to avoid the pressure on his mouth. But a trainer teaching a horse to be bridle-wise does more than simply use the bit. If he wishes the horse to turn left, he also lays the right-hand rein against the horse's neck and indicates by the pressure of his knee that he wants the horse to turn. After a while, the horse will turn left at rein touch and knee pressure even though the bit has not been used. A good bridle-wise horse can be ridden with a halter, being completely "cued" by the reins and knees of his rider, although originally these cues meant nothing to him.

It is true that horses can be forced to go through certain routines by the constant threat of punishment, but the system sooner or later is sure to backfire. A trainer once told me a story that is a good illustration of this.

"Harold, my oldest boy, was offered a very fine dressage horse by an old-time trainer who believed in treating his horses rough. This horse could do a pas-et-un-sault [leap straight up with all four feet clear of the ground], the Spanish March [throw up the forelegs with each step], and a two-step [going forward and to one side at the same time, the front and hind legs crossing]. Harold tried out the horse in the practice ring. The horse did perfectly and Harold couldn't figure out why the man wanted to get rid of him. But he found out quickly enough when he tried working the animal in a show. The horse balked and wouldn't do a thing. It took us some time to figure out what was the matter. We learned that the old trainer used to beat the horse to make him perform, using a short length of chain so it wouldn't leave marks as a whip does. The horse was smart enough to find out that the man didn't dare beat him in a show ring where there were a lot of people around, so he would balk in a show and work all right in practice. When Harold found that out, he took along a six-inch length of chain in his pocket when he exhibited the horse. When he started to balk, Harold would rattle the chain. Instantly the horse's ears would shoot up and he'd work perfectly. But we got rid of that animal. We knew that after a while he'd catch on to the chain-rattling gag and refuse to work."

Horses live in a world of scent as well as sight and sound. A good trainer never forgets this. A highly experienced trainer explained how he taught four horses to run a race while each was being ridden by a different animal. The animal jockeys were a leopard, a monkey, a bear, and a dog. Several men had tried to train the horses by putting blinders on them so they couldn't see their animal riders. This plan hadn't worked. The horses could smell the animals on their backs and the strange odor drove them crazy. So the trainer started off by keeping each horse tied near the pen of the animal that was to ride him. After a few days, the horse got accustomed to the animal's scent. Then the horse's head was covered with a leather shield and the animal put on his back. When the horse grew accustomed to the strange rider, the shield was removed.

As with lion trainers, horse trainers like to take advantage of some trait in a horse's nature that can be built up into a trick. This is especially true in motion picture work, where it is often necessary to have a "fighting horse" that will rear and lash out with his forelegs when a man approaches him (usually to defend his beloved master from the villainous cattle rustlers). The trainer starts out by purchasing a naturally aggressive horse, generally a yearling colt that has been mishandled and learned that he can frighten people by attacking them. Formerly, the trainer's most difficult job was transporting the colt to the trainer's stable without using force, because once the horse learned that the man was unafraid and could make him obey, the colt came to respect the man and lost much of his aggressiveness. Now tranquilizers are used. The colt is then put in a small corral with a lunge line on him and the trainer approaches him bent over. Suddenly the man straightens up, shouts, and waves his hands. That encourages the horse to rear and strike at him. The man instantly retreats, leaving the horse alone. Soon the colt becomes convinced that he has everyone bluffed and will attack anyone approaching him. Eventually, the colt's rearing becomes automatic and loses all its original aggressiveness. He can then be handled like any other horse.

I have seen a horse trained to pick up a coin in his mouth, walk over to a cash register, ring the bell, open the drawer, put the coin in, and then close the drawer. He could also open a window, climb through, and finally walk over a pair of lovers while giving them a "horse laugh." The trainer wouldn't tell me how he was about to teach a horse such a routine. "I've got to have some secrets," he explained, "or everybody would be a trainer." Again, this is a wonderful example of what horses can be taught to do with proper handling.

All horses do not necessarily respond to the same methods. Some will shake their heads for "no" if they are tapped on a certain spot on the withers with the blunt end of a pencil; others won't respond to this stimulus and the trainer has to blow in the horse's ear. Some horses will nod if the trainer tickles their chins;

others will nod only if you keep tapping them on the chest. Some horses won't learn tricks at all. You have to have good material to work with.

Many tricks require elaborate step-by-step training. A favorite trick is to have the hero tied up by the villians, then his faithful horse appears and unties him with his teeth. The trainer usually begins by getting the horse to pick up a handkerchief by wrapping a bit of apple in it. The horse smells the apple and shakes the cloth to get it out. Eventually, the horse will pick up any cloth he sees and shake it, hoping to find some apple. Then the trainer substitutes a short length of rope. As the horse is now accustomed to picking up any object the trainer indicates, he picks up the rope. He is instantly rewarded with a bit of apple. Finally, the horse learns to untie the rope and bring it to his trainer for an apple reward.

Sometimes a trainer's solution to what seems an insoluble problem is very simple. There was a big rosinback with the circus who was so nervous that whenever the audience laughed or applauded, he panicked. Short of tranquilizing him before each performance, there seemed to be no answer to the problem. Then an old-time trainer intervened.

"Give me five minutes alone with that horse, and he'll be all right," the man promised. Man and horse withdrew. When they returned, the horse went through the entire routine without trouble.

"Are you really sure you didn't tranquilize him?" I asked the trainer doubtfully.

"Sure I'm sure. I just put cotton in his ears so he couldn't hear the noise," the man explained casually.

Horses often develop close attachments to a stable mate, so close in fact that if they are separated, the horse left behind goes nearly mad. I was told of a trainer who was called to Hollywood because none of the regular trainers there were able to arrange for a certain scene in which a horse who had joined a herd of wild mustangs was supposed to leave the bunch and run toward the hero when he heard his master's voice. As horses are very herd-conscious, it was found impossible to get a horse to leave the others. At one point, the studio even had a length of piano wire tied around the horse's neck and pulled him out of the herd by sheer strength. The trouble with this was that the horse approached his beloved master with all four feet firmly planted in front of him, obviously fighting every step of the way.

The circus trainer had two horses that were stable mates and much attached to each other. He took them to Hollywood and one was turned loose with the studio herd. The trainer held the other behind the actor, just out of camera range. When the trainer's held horse saw his friend, he whinnied loudly. At once, his friend left the herd and ran toward him. In the picture, it seemed as though he were running eagerly toward the actor.

However, even the best of trainers make mistakes. One man was asked by Mrs. Buck Jones to train a horse for her husband for a surprise Christmas present. Although the public likes to think that cowboy stars train their own horses, this is seldom the case. The trainer spent weeks working on a fine pinto gelding, and delivered the horse to the Jones home on Christmas Eve. There were a number of prominent motion picture people in the living room and Mrs. Jones thought it would be a nice idea to have the horse go over to Buck and make a one-knee bow. The trainer showed her how to cue the pinto for this trick and then left.

When he returned to his hotel, he found that Mrs. Jones had been telephoning him desperately for the last half hour. The trainer called her back and asked anxiously, "Wouldn't the horse make the bow?"

"Oh, he made the bow all right," Mrs. Jones assured him. "But there's just one thing I forgot to ask you. How the heck do you cue the darned animal to straighten up again so we can get him out of the room?"

The last time the circus played Philly, I was called in just before tear-down to check some of the animals. Afterwards, I went to the station to see them off. Nearly everyone knew me and many were shouting, "Come on, Dr. Lose, come with us. We need a vet now that old Doc Henderson has retired. There's a bunk for you. Join the show!"

You know, I was tempted. I really was. They're such nice

people and traveling around the country would be a change from my usual veterinary work. For a minute there, I nearly threw my bag on board the train and jumped in after it. But of course I couldn't; I had too many responsibilities here. I could only laugh, shake my head, and wave as the train pulled away.

9

WITH THE
MOUNTED POLICE

FOR YEARS I HAD BEEN DREAMING ABOUT BUILDING MY OWN equine hospital. The closest was at New Bolton Center, University of Pennsylvania School of Veterinary Medicine, over 30 miles away. Besides, I had a number of ideas that I wanted to see incorporated in a hospital for horses. My practice had grown; in addition to handling the DuPont and Biddle stables, I was now first veterinarian for the Pancoast and Lyman stables as well as for numerous smaller establishments. Busy as I was, there was no chance for me to raise enough money to build a private hospital. However, at one time it had seemed impossible that I would ever get to be a veterinarian at all, so I knew miracles could happen.

The miracle happened at two o'clock one morning when I was getting in after a hard day and found Audrey Bostwick sitting in our living room surrounded by empty coffee cups. "Where on earth have you been?" she started. "Norma, your mother, and I have been trying to locate you since seven. They gave up and went to bed, but I decided you'd have to get in sometime unless you were dead and the police promised to call me if they found your body. They didn't call so I figured you were all right."

I poured myself a cup of coffee and fell into a chair. "All right," I said wearily. "What's the emergency?"

"You're the new veterinarian for the Philadelphia Mounted Police," she told me. "One hundred horses. With your regular practice, that should keep you busy."

I tried to think of some witty comeback to this heavy-handed joke. Dr. McCarthy was the police veterinarian and I knew the department was well satisfied with him. In any case, the police veterinarian had always been a man. Furthermore, an outgoing veterinarian always has a great deal to say about his successor, and I knew that Dr. McCarthy had a poor opinion of me. Once when Inspector Turner had called me in to treat a horse's infected gums, Dr. McCarthy was furious that a woman had been consulted.

"Have I got time to drink this coffee before I take on my new duties?" was the best that I could do.

Audrey looked at me hard. "Barely. Drink it, then start writing up your list of qualifications. I'll take it back with me to Philadelphia when I go. Dr. McCarthy has just retired. There's the little formality that the police commissioners have got to approve you."

I didn't know whether to be delighted or shocked. I was already carrying a heavy schedule. There were four police stables, all scattered around Philadelphia, which was 40 miles from Berwyn. Most of my practice lay west of the Main Line, in the opposite direction from Philly. I also knew that in police work, you had to be ready to attend an emergency at any hour of the day and night, and there were plenty of emergencies. Still, it was a great honor. As far as I knew, I would be the first woman police veterinarian in history. I liked the police and they seemed to like me. And there was my dreamed-of hospital. This would give me the chance to build it.

I drew up my list of qualifications and Audrey left with it. She was a great deal more confident than I. On thinking it over, I decided that the whole idea had been Audrey's rather than the police commissioners', so I pretty much forgot about it.

A week later, I was called to appear before the commissioners who would examine me. I got a brand-new set of coveralls, made sure my shoes were shined, and drove to Philadelphia. The commissioners gave me a rather strict examination, which I was lucky enough to pass. It lasted for two hours, part written and

167

part oral. They seemed particularly interested in my educational background and in the fact that I had worked almost exclusively with horses rather than with animals in general. As I was signing the contract, one of them remarked: "Oh yes, you'll also be taking care of the seventeen German Shepherd police dogs. Be careful of them. They're killers."

I hadn't counted on this. I'm not at my best with dogs. Still there was no help for it now.

I thought that I had been busy before. Now I felt as though I'd been on a vacation. As part of my regular practice, I had to supervise a large breeding farm near Downingtown, a good 50 miles from Philadelphia. Since I regarded working with pregnant mares and delivering foals as my specialty, I had to spend much of my time there. Every morning I left the house at five o'clock, and I mean every morning—Sundays and Christmas too, and I had to go, well or sick. I would check all the police stables first, then go on to the breeding farm. From there I went to a second breeding farm near Unionville, 30 miles in another direction. Then my usual rounds. In the evenings, I checked the police stables again. Of course, I was constantly in touch with Mother and Norma by car radio so that, in case of an emergency, I could interrupt my usual rounds to answer the call.

My first problem was with the dogs. By definition, an attack dog isn't a household pet. Many of them wouldn't permit anyone to handle them except their master. Several had to be put in a squeeze cage—with movable sides that can be slid inward to hold the animal motionless for treatment. I felt as though I were back in the circus with the wild animals. Luckily, the dogs were a healthy lot so I had little to do except vaccinate and worm them. I know that many people feel a certain resentment toward the police for using dogs in their work; much of this feeling, I believe, is an atavism of the days when human beings were threatened by wolves. Often people are more frightened of an animal than an armed man, even though an officer with a gun or a heavy nightstick is far more dangerous than any dog. Yet on several occasions I have seen men who were prepared to attack armed police officers turn and run from a snarling, growling dog. The advantage in using dogs is to overtake a fugitive running down a dark alley or dodging in and out among parked cars. A policeman is at a great disadvantage in such a situation; he does not know if the fugitive is armed and may suddenly turn and fire at him. A dog is smaller than a man, faster, and quicker. He can bring the fugitive to bay and hold him until the officer comes up. Of course, police dogs can be misused, as I believe they were in certain southern cities during the race riots of twenty years ago; but so for that matter can firearms, clubs, or fire hoses.

I might add here that police dogs attack only on command; they do not decide whom to attack. Even so, in my experience they are animals very much better left alone. I hate to see people go over and try to pet them. They are on duty and dislike being bothered. Except when turned loose to attack, they are always kept on a leash, which is most wise. Anyway, nearly all my duties were with the horses—thankfully.

I had taken for granted that my work with police horses would be pretty much like my work in private stables. I soon found out how wrong I was.

I remember I was driving along Lincoln Pike once late in the afternoon with Barbara. Suddenly the radio crackled and Norma's voice came over it with an emergency call: "A mounted policeman and his horse have fallen over a cliff into Wissahickon Creek. The man has gotten clear but the horse is in quicksand and sinking. Get there fast!"

I couldn't imagine how I could get a horse out of quicksand. After he was free, perhaps I might be of help. But this was no time to argue.

"Where exactly is the horse?" I asked.

"Go to Bells Mill Road. There's a police car waiting there to guide you. Don't worry about the speed limit. Tie a white handkerchief to your radio antenna and drive as fast as you can. Any policeman who sees you will know it's an emergency."

Barbara instantly had the window open and was tying the handkerchief in place as I stepped on the accelerator. It was a wild ride. As we approached Bells Mill Road, I saw the police car waiting. When he saw us, he instantly switched on his flashing light and with his siren screaming, started off. I followed him as closely as I could. Wissahickon Creek is a surprisingly wild section of country on the northwestern fringe of the city. The creek itself is really a small river, especially in flood time, and we had had heavy rains that spring; it flows along the base of a cliff that in places is perhaps 100 feet high. The whole area is heavily wooded with only a few bridle paths leading through it. We tore along the outskirts at top speed.

The police car skidded to a stop where a crowd had collected, all seemingly intent on something deep in the woods. There were a number of policemen who quickly cleared a way for us through the mob. I had my black bag and Barbara followed carrying whatever odds and ends she thought we might need. Suddenly we found ourselves on the edge of what appeared to be a precipice.

A police chief, an old friend, was in charge. As soon as he saw us, he shouted over the cliff: "The vet's here with her helper. Get ready!" I heard voices coming from below, and the next instant Barbara and I were led to the brink of the sheer drop. Heights have never been in my line and it was growing dark. I could see no way down and I admit that I was scared stiff.

Barbara must have sensed it for she said, "Give me the bag, Doctor. That'll leave you both hands free."

"No, I'll take it with me," I said, in what I hoped was a firm voice.

Now I could see that a human chain of police was stationed at intervals on the cliff's face. How they hung on I have no idea, but each had obviously found a handhold. The topmost man stretched up one hand for me while holding onto the root of a tree with the other. My legs were trembling, the pit of my stomach felt as though I'd swallowed a pound of ice, and the muscles in my throat were stiff as wires. Still, I managed to take the extended hand and slide over the edge. Holding onto the bag with one hand, I slipped down the side, trying to dig in with my heels. The second policeman a little lower grabbed me and although my additional weight nearly dislodged him, I managed to make it to the third man. Above me I could hear Barbara coming. I wondered what would happen if she lost her footing and came down on top of me. We would both have ended up at the bottom with broken bones if not broken necks. Fortunately, Barbara was more sure-footed than I and hardly needed the men's help.

At last we came to the bottom, by the creek's bank. I felt like falling down on the level ground in relief but there was no time.

A boat was ready with four men at the oars and several more holding the boat against the bank, for the creek was swollen and it was all they could do to keep the craft from being carried downstream. When Barbara and I climbed aboard, our combined weights brought the boat so low in the water that there was barely an inch of freeboard. The men let go instantly and we were swept downstream, the men pulling at the oars hardly able to guide us.

The creek is full of rocks and between them ran white water rapids; we rushed along like a roller coaster. I had often seen the creek in daylight and it had seemed a peaceful stream, one you could wade across without too much trouble. Now it was a dangerous torrent. If we turned over, we would be sucked down into the boiling water and I seriously doubted if we could make it to land. The boat was shipping water rapidly and I sat holding my black bag high to keep the contents dry, wondering where the horse could be and how he and his rider had ever come to fall over the cliff.

Luckily, we had only a few hundred yards to go before the rowers forced us into a backwater. There was a quagmire about 100 feet square composed of black sticky mud and green scum. In the center was the poor horse, a big gelding I recognized as Major, one of the best horses in the corps. Major was a splendid animal with a proud way of walking, but there was nothing proud about him now. He was hopelessly mired in the morass, barely able to move his head which, together with a portion of his back, was all that showed. There was no sign of his rider.

My first thought was to get to the trapped animal and give him a sedative, as horses often die from shock less serious than what he had been through. I tried to crawl across the mud but sank in too deeply.

"Has anyone an ax?" I shouted. "Cut down some branches and make a mat across this mud that will hold me."

Now I heard more sirens and saw fire engines in the distance. *They must have the whole police force plus the fire department here,* I thought. I was very nearly right. Used to the show rings and racetracks where so many people tend to regard horses as simply a commodity to be bought and sold, I had forgotten the intense empathy that exists between the mounted police and their chargers. Just as policemen are intensely loyal to each other—the worst mistake a criminal can make is to injure a policeman—so they also feel a strong bond toward their horses. If a horse is in trouble, the whole department turns out to help.

The cliff ended several hundred yards from where we were but the fire engines could not reach us because of the trees. However, half a dozen men soon appeared with axes and began cutting limbs. Meanwhile, Barbara had tried to wiggle out to Major by spreading herself flat on the ooze, but then she too had to give up. The men started throwing down branches and covering them with blankets. Finally, I was able to inch my way over the squashy bridge and reach Major.

Major weighed 1,400 pounds and was hopelessly mired. He could no longer keep his head up and it had fallen into the mud. I gave him an injection to keep him going and shouted to Barbara to help me. She had already started across the branches and blankets with an intravenous injection needle and bottle. Slowly, he began to revive.

"Get ropes and pass them under him!" I shouted, for with his new strength Major had begun to struggle again and this was sending him deeper into the muck. Now we had another problem. The blanket bridge was too weak to support the weight of men in addition to Barbara and myself, yet we didn't dare stop the I.V. injections. Finally, while Barbara held the I.V. bottle and needle, I was able to take the ropes passed out to me by the firemen and get them under Major's body.

Thirty men heaved on each rope. When they felt Major move, they started cheering. I could see Major react to the sound. He had begun to slump again, but now he picked up spirit. "Keep on cheering!" I shouted. Slowly they dragged Major closer and closer to the edge of the creek. If he began to struggle now, he would go into the racing water and be carried away. Three of the men on the lines did get sucked into the stream and had to be taken to the hospital, half-drowned. But gradually we were able to get Major to the solid ground and on his feet. When I shouted, "He's out!" a great shout went up and the men around me called to the others further away, "He's out!" We could hear them cheering.

Major was shaking and in a bad state of shock. He was unable to walk and for a few moments it seemed as though all our efforts had been useless. Then men appeared with power saws and cut a path through the trees along which the police horse ambulance was able to make its way. Meanwhile, we wrapped Major in dry blankets. Between the blankets and the sedation we were injecting in him, he stopped shaking.

Despite everything the men could do, the ambulance couldn't quite reach him. With men supporting him on each side and Barbara and me at his head, we were able to get him to move forward step by step until he saw the ambulance. Major had ridden in it before and he recognized it as meaning safety. With a whinny, he reeled forward, pricking up his ears. We loaded him in without trouble. I rode in the van with him to the hospital, still fearful of a relapse, but Major was now quite all right. At the hospital a warm bath and, an hour later, a meal of hot bran mash was all he needed. He had recovered by the next day and put in several more years on the force.

How had he ever happened to fall off the cliff? His rider had been on patrol in the park when he heard a woman scream. He turned Major off the bridle path and galloped through the trees toward the sound. He saw several men running away and took after them. As the men vanished among the trees, the officer crashed through the brush after them—and horse and man went over the cliff. They hit the water some distance apart. When the man came up, it was all he could do to keep afloat in the rapids. He made it to solid ground, but poor Major had got mired down in the quicksand. The officer stumbled through the woods until he came to a road and was able to hail a passing car. No one ever found out who the woman was who had screamed or what became of the men molesting her.

Philadelphia has always been especially proud of its mounted police. In wooded areas like Wissahickon Park they are crucially important, for cars cannot get into many sections and a man on foot goes too slowly. The mounted police have many other uses, too. In case of city disturbances, a mounted policeman can see over the heads of a crowd and spot the troublemakers. He can also follow a fugitive down narrow alleys. I have always felt that people are more impressed by a mounted man than a police car. Last year when the Philadelphia hockey team, the Fliers, won the Stanley Cup, the returning heroes touched off a near riot. I was there and it was most impressive to see the skill both men and horses showed in handling a mob that at times got completely out of hand and was actually a menace. I am sure men on foot or in cars could not possibly have done the job. The mounted police drill team gives exhibitions at fairs, horse shows, and festivals that are most impressive and excellent public relations for the police force.

When I became police veterinarian, the mounted corps consisted of only seventy horses; in 1970, Mayor Rizzo added another hundred horses and men to the force. This really kept me racing from one stable to another. A new stable was built at Belmont with stalls for one hundred horses, and an inside and outside ring. The inside ring had movable walls which swung open on pivots that could let in air and light on good days but stay shut in bad weather. It also had large mirrors mounted on the sides so the men could see themselves as they rode past and correct their mistakes. All this was magnificent but a lot of work. Much of my time was spent checking the horses' hoofs and special shoes, which took heavy punishment on the hard city streets. It was very different indeed from treating saddle horses and thoroughbreds on their country estates.

A major problem was finding horses suitable for police duty. They had to be big animals, quiet and capable of going for long hours without rest. The corps got a few from upstate in the Pennsylvania Dutch country where horses are still the standard means of work and transportation, but the animals offered for sale were usually old, sick, or had some vice that made them unsuitable. Whenever I heard of a horse sale anywhere on the East Coast, I told Inspector Turner and he sent a man to pick up any horses that would make good chargers.

One day in late summer, I was called to the Belmont stables by a puzzled police sergeant. "Dr. Lose, a horse just walked in here and refuses to leave. Right now he's drinking at the watering trough. He's pretty badly cut up and I wish you'd look at him."

"Hasn't he any tack on him?" I wanted to know.

"Not even a halter. He isn't shod, either. He's a fine, big chestnut gelding about seventeen hands but in very poor shape. Even in his present condition, I'd say he's worth several hundred dollars at least. We haven't any idea where he came from or who owns him."

I thought rapidly. There wasn't a privately owned stable anywhere in the vicinity of Belmont. There had been no horse shows, rodeos, or circuses in Philadelphia for weeks. If anyone had been missing a horse, he would surely have notified the police, and no horse would be kept unshod and without a halter in this locality. Horses just don't wander around loose without attracting some attention; they're too big.

"I'll be right over," I said.

Norma went with me, as she was equally curious to see the animal. When we arrived, the horse had a crowd around him. The sergeant had wisely put a halter on him and led him away from the watering trough as he had been drinking so heavily he might have foundered himself.

He was indeed in wretched shape. He had a number of lacerations and his legs were swollen as though he had walked a long way on hard streets. He was also pitifully thin. I had the men wash him off with warm water. He had several bruises but his legs were the most seriously injured. I cleaned out his cuts, sutured the worst places, and put antiseptic bandages around his sore legs. I also gave injections to prevent infection and a booster to prevent lockjaw.

"He'll be all right," I told the sergeant, and looking at him, I knew we were both thinking the same thing. The chestnut was just the sort of horse the police needed; but, of course, even though he had been neglected and wandering around loose, every effort would have to be made to locate the rightful owner.

In a few weeks, the stranger had recovered sufficiently to be ridden. A crowd collected in the paddock to watch. So far no word had come from the owner, although a description of the chestnut had been run in the newspapers and all dealers notified. Personally, I suspected the animal was probably incurably vicious, which was why his master had turned him loose and now refused to admit ownership. One of the corps' best riders tacked him up, then mounted him. Everyone waited for an explosion, but the horse stood quietly until the rider clucked to him and shook the reins. The chestnut moved off at a steady walk. After taking him once around the ring, the rider had him trot and canter. As far as we could tell, he was gentle and well broken.

"Why should anyone abandon a horse like that?" asked the sergeant. "And why in the middle of a city?" We discussed it for the next half hour but no one had even a theory.

"Legally, we can't keep him without a transfer of ownership, signed by the owner," the sergeant said at last. "But we can't just turn him loose again, that's for sure. We'll keep him as a charger so he can earn his keep. Of course, if the real owner turns up we'll have to let him go. It's too bad because he's the sort of horse we need and everyone in the stable likes him. I'm going to call him Traveler because he sure must have come a long way."

So Traveler stayed on at the Belmont stables. He not only made an excellent police horse, he proved so capable that he joined the exclusive drill team. He had filled out, his legs were in good condition, and his wounds had healed without leaving any scars. Everyone was proud of him.

Then came disaster. One afternoon, an old jalopy drove up to the Belmont stables. A heavyset man wearing blue jeans and a cowboy hat walked into the office and asked, "You heard anything about a chestnut horse I lost a couple of months ago? I figured somebody might have seen him."

I was sent for. The sergeant, Inspector Turner, and the officer who was Traveler's rider all questioned the man closely. There was no doubt the horse he was describing was Traveler.

The man was a dealer and had been driving a truck loaded with horses across the state. While on the Schuylkill Expressway, the rear door of the truck had come open and Traveler had fallen out of the moving vehicle. Why he wasn't killed or at least suffered a broken leg I'll never know. But the horse had managed to survive, crossed the crowded turnpike, and after wandering about in the wooded areas of Fairmount Park at last smelled the other horses at Belmont and headed for the stables. When his owner had finally discovered him missing, he had taken his other horses to the sale, disposed of them, and was now back-tracking in the hopes of finding the missing horse.

Unfortunately, we made a bad mistake We let the man see Traveler. Instead of the sickly, weak animal he had lost, here was a magnificent horse in prime condition and obviously well trained. The dealer was astonished and delighted. "Well, I will say you took good care of him," he admitted. "I'll be takin' him along now."

The horse was legally his, no doubt about it. I knew it, Inspector Turner knew it, all the men at the stables knew it.

"Will you sell him?" asked Inspector Turner.

Yes, the man was willing to part with Traveler, although he admitted it would be a terrible wrench. He named a price. You could have gotten Citation for the same money.

Then I had one of my rare inspirations. "The police department can't afford that," I explained, "so you'd better take the horse. Oh yes, before you do there's my bill for veterinary services over the last two months, plus drugs and medicines. Then, naturally, there's his board and stable fees. It comes to a total of . . ." and I reeled off a figure that would have given even Mr. Biddle or Mrs. DuPont pause.

It ended by the department getting Traveler for a reasonable sum. He went on to distinguish himself with the drill team. When not with the team, he worked everywhere from crowded central city to the bridle paths of the parks. He was one of the best chargers I have ever seen.

As I said earlier, the French have a rather unfortunate saying, "The only trustworthy horse is a dead horse." Being fond of horses, I don't care for this proverb. Yet I will say that horses are highly individualistic and no one can claim that he knows what a horse will do. I like to think that I can usually size one up fairly well, but there are times I've been fooled. This has happened several times with the police chargers, partly because they live and work under such different conditions from thoroughbreds or ordinary riding horses.

The corps acquired a beautiful horse named Sansirmac. Sansirmac was an English stallion and had been a racehorse. He had won over $160,000 on the turf, then strained a tendon. He had always been a temperamental animal; in fact, he was vicious, and his reputation was such that his owner decided not to keep him as a stud, so he presented him to the police department. Frankly, it was the sort of present the department could have done without although Sansirmac was a valuable animal. He was so handsome that the men were determined to use him if possible. I was called in to check him and give him the standard vaccine injections.

I took one look at the big animal with his ears laid back, the whites of his eyes showing, and his teeth bared, and said, "Put a nose twitch on him—if you can." Four men went into the stall to handle the thoroughbred. The horse knocked one man over the lower part of the double door, two others managed to escape over the top of the stall, and the fourth was badly trampled. They finally got the twitch on him and I gave him the injections. When I left, I told them, "Take my advice and get rid of that animal. He's incurably mean, and a menace. There's a good chance he may kill someone."

But the stable sergeant wouldn't take my advice; the horse was so stunning he refused to part with him. As far as looks went, he was by far the handsomest horse in the corps. So I only said, "Keep the stall door locked. If one of the stablemen goes in by mistake, he'll be lucky to come out alive."

A mistake was made and the stall was left open. A few days later, a raw rookie who had just joined the force and knew absolutely nothing about horses was walking down the aisle of the stable. He was attracted by Sansirmac's looks, opened the stall door, and went in. With the confidence of ignorance, he walked over, patted the horse, stroked his neck, and stood admiring him. Sansirmac sniffed at him but made no other move. Then the rookie had another idea. He got a saddle and a bridle and tried to tack up the thoroughbred. He had only the vaguest idea how to go about it, but Sansirmac stood like a rocking horse while the man put on the tack, all wrong end to, and then clumsily mounted. A little later, the sergeant happened to walk past the paddock and stopped appalled. There was the rookie, trotting Sansirmac around the ring, bouncing up and down in the saddle in a way calculated to drive the gentlest horse crazy. Sansirmac, however, was doing everything in his power to make up for his rider's ineptitude. When the Sergeant hurried forward to grab the thoroughbred's bridle, Sansirmac furiously attacked him.

From then on, Sansirmac was the rookie's horse. As long as the man was with him, Sansirmac was beautifully behaved. He even learned to tolerate other people—if the rookie was with him. After a spell in the parks, he was put on the central city beat. Because of the noise, crowds, and heavy vehicular traffic, few horses can stand this beat, but Sansirmac did splendidly. Then came the climax, as far as I was concerned. At Christmas, the rookie dressed up as Santa Claus and with a sack full of toys and loudly jangling bells that would have driven an ordinary horse up the wall rode through the back streets distributing presents to the children who crowded around him, patting the horse, pulling his tail, and getting under his feet. Sansirmac took it all calmly.

There is only one person Sansirmac still won't tolerate even when under the control of his beloved rider, who incidentally is now no longer a rookie but an accomplished horseman. That person is me. Sansirmac remembers well that it was I who stuck a needle into him, and whenever I go near his stall, he tries to murder me. He is the hardest horse to treat I've ever seen. I pray that his health stays good!

Why did Sansirmac allow the rookie to handle him in the first place? I have occasionally seen vicious horses who will allow a child to do anything with them when they would attack an adult. Frankly I don't know why this is. I can only suppose that the horse senses the innocence of the child and his utter absence of fear. It must have been the rookie's childlike approach that quieted Sansirmac. Although I have known horses to behave like this, I wouldn't count on it. No child, or inexperienced adult either for that matter, should be allowed near a potentially dangerous horse.

In stark contrast to the belligerent Sansirmac, there was Huey. Huey was a big gelding, powerful, reasonably intelligent, and the biggest coward I've ever seen. He was terrified of dogs or even cats. If one walked past him, Huey stood shaking with fear. If a car backfired, Huey nearly fainted. Because he was so extremely gentle he was used for city patrol work, as Huey would never resent anything done to him and there was no chance that he would kick or bite anyone even when struck or beaten—as I regret to say police chargers occasionally are by unthinking or cruel people. I liked Huey, as did everyone who knew him; still I

179

was afraid that sometime a situation would arise where Huey would be called on to show some determination, and Huey had no more spirit than a canary. Not as much.

One evening, Huey and his rider were patrolling a part of the city known as a high-crime area. Suddenly there were shouts, a shot, and a man appeared running for his life, followed by a second man brandishing a pistol. Huey's rider put spurs to him and Huey galloped in pursuit, not realizing of course that he was taking part in a potentially dangerous situation. As soon as he saw the mounted policeman, the gunman turned and ran in another direction while his intended victim collapsed in a doorway. Huey's rider took off after the gunman. The man quickly found he could not outdistance the horseman and turned at bay, aiming his pistol at the officer. Only a few yards separated them and the officer found himself looking down the barrel of the loaded weapon. There was no way he could avoid the bullet. He was as good as dead. But at that very instant the always nervous Huey took fright at the sight of the gunman's lifted arm and reared just as the man fired. The bullet hit Huey in the neck. As he went down, a police car dashed up and the would-be assassin was arrested.

I was making my rounds when Mother called me on the car radio and told me what had happened to poor Huey. I had my niece Margaret with me at the time, who fortunately is a trained surgical assistant. As usual when anything happens to a horse, every officer felt personally involved. Orders went out from headquarters to adjust the traffic lights so I wouldn't have to stop. I roared through the city at top speed to the back street where Huey was lying semi-conscious on the cobblestones, his rider sitting beside him trying to stop the beeding. The horse ambulance arrived at almost the same time. With the help of several officers, we were able to get Huey on his feet and into the van where, as he could not stand, he was supported by a belly band. Then we started off for the hospital, two police cars leading with their lights flashing and traffic officers stopping traffic in all directions as we went by. When we reached the hospital, I found that Huey could not walk; he could barely stand and was losing quantities of blood.

Two men got on either side of him, clasping hands under his

body to support him. Inch by inch the belly band was slackened while Huey shook so from shock and fright the whole van trembled. Now came the crucial moment. To unload him, he had to be turned around. Gradually the men worked him around while Barbara and I strove to stop the hemorrhaging. Then three men stood on the van's ramp to receive him while two more hung onto his tail to keep him from plunging forward too rapidly. Slowly he was taken off the van, and then by sheer manpower carried to the hospital. If he had gone down that would have been that, for it was impossible for the men to lift him. By a great show of strength and determination, the officers got him into a stall and then piled bales of hay beside him to keep him on his feet.

Now everything was up to Margaret and me. I even called Norma into duty. I gave Huey a sedative and injected a local anesthetic where a trickle of blood was coming from the bullet wound. We covered him with a porous wool cooler because his body temperature had dropped sharply from shock and loss of blood. Then we started getting intravenous fluids into him. Margaret brought up our portable X-ray apparatus and I tried to find the location of the bullet. There are so many planes in a horse's neck that this was a tediously long job requiring many, many views. We were in the middle of it when we heard the door open and men's voices shouting: "Roll the cameras up here! Look out for the end of that stall—somebody hit the lights!"

"What's all this?" I demanded.

Television crews had arrived. A man I suppose was the director came up to me.

"This horse is a hero! He threw up his head to take the bullet meant for his rider. The police commissioner is going to have a special medal struck in his honor—for conspicuous courage. He's receiving a special citation; only time in history a horse has gotten such a thing. It's going to be front-page news all over the country." I quietly but firmly ordered them out.

Good old Huey! Still, if he was going to survive to receive his medal, I'd have to find the bullet fast.

I probed the wound in his neck gently. As the forceps were inserted, I could hear air escaping through the opening. That meant that either the trachea or the windpipe had been penetrated. Now I would have to find out whether the bullet had dropped down the trachea into the lungs or passed through the trachea and was in the tissue of Huey's neck.

Swelling had begun to interfere with the passage of air—Huey's breathing was becoming labored. Margaret hurried to the surgical prep room and returned with a compact surgical pack. Huey's neck was scrubbed and shaved and a tracheotomy tube slipped into the wound. He took a deep breath and air rushed through the tube into his lungs. The relief he felt was instantly apparent; he began to breathe easily.

Again my staff and I used the portable X-ray. The first pictures through the rapid automatic developer showed a tiny light area at the edge of one of the films that might possibly be the small bullet. More X-ray pictures showed the bullet clearly. It was lodged against the spinal column in an angle formed by the bony process and the body of the vertebra. Because of the small caliber of the gun the force of the bullet had caused no damage to the skeletal structures, but the position was precarious. It had to be removed.

To locate and remove a bullet deeply embedded in muscle tissue and adjacent to many intertwining nerves without inflicting damage to the soft nerve fibers and tissues is a delicate operation. It took me three and a half hours, helped by Margaret my nurse (or) Nancy Norma, and my anesthesiologist Dr. Franchetti. At last Huey slept on a foam-rubber mattress and I put the bullet in a special plastic envelope that sealed with a tamper-proof flap. I also signed a statement to the effect that the bullet had come from Huey's neck, with the date and time, and that only I had handled it. The envelope was picked up by the Crime Detection Laboratory to be used in evidence against the gunman, who was convicted of attempted murder.

Huey recovered and resumed his duties. He became known as the "hero horse" and appeared on television, in the newspapers, and magazines. I have grown very much attached to him and only hope that he doesn't drop dead from heart failure if he meets a belligerent rabbit someday.

Not all police horse stories had such happy endings. Being a policeman is a high-risk profession and I am afraid the same can be said of their horses. The danger does not always come from gunmen nor even, more commonly, from drunk or reckless drivers. The work of a policeman—or his charger—is not limited to the detection of crime. An officer must be ready to handle any emergency and his charger is supposed to do the same.

One afternoon after a violent thunderstorm, I got a call on the car radio to go once to the corner of 63rd and the Parkway to treat a horse that had collapsed. I remember that the traffic was terrible. Several of the roads were flooded, which meant that all cars had been shunted onto the few good highways. As usual, there was a police car waiting for me, and with siren and flashing lights it guided me around the worst places. Then we came to a standstill. There was a hopeless jam of police cars, private cars, for me, I managed to get through the mob. Ahead of me, I saw and crowds of people. With two policemen running interference where wires were down and near them lay the body of Jo-Jo, a fine chestnut gelding with white stockings. He was one of our best horses. What a waste! His rider stood a few yards off, openly and unashamedly crying.

I started toward them when a dozen voices shouted: "Look out—those are live wires! The ground's charged with electricity!"

I stopped dead. Everywhere were pools of water, the wires lying in them. I circled the area and asked the sobbing officer, "What happened?"

He said in a choked voice, "Jo-Jo and I were riding our beat and I saw the wires were down. The road was blocked ahead and people were getting out of their cars and wandering around. I shouted to them to keep back and Jo-Jo trotted to head them off. As he went past that light there, he fell down as though he'd been shot. The wet ground and his steel shoes carried the current right through him. I could feel the charge in my hands where they held the reins. All that saved me was my saddle; it was new, dry, and heavily padded. I tried to drop the reins but the current constricted my muscles and I couldn't let go. At last I jumped as far as I could. I must have just been able to get clear of the charged area for my hands opened and I was all right. But Jo-Jo's dead."

I was sure he was right but I said, "There may still be life in him. As soon as the current is shut off, I'll go and see."

I never saw such a mess. People were coming from all directions, attracted by the excitement and ignorant of the danger. Then with a howling of sirens, the TV trucks came tearing up. One thing was sure. Poor Jo-Jo hadn't given his life in vain. If it hadn't been for him, a number of people, especially children, as it was near a playground, would have been killed sloshing through the electrified wet ground. People either ignored the wires or thought that as long as they didn't touch them, they were safe. They didn't realize that the whole area for a distance of 20 or 30 yards was a deathtrap.

Then Inspector Turner arrived and told me that the electric company had turned off the current, so it was now safe to go in. But he insisted on going in first and touching the horse to make sure there was no danger. I followed him with Jo-Jo's rider right after me. I hardly needed my stethoscope to tell that Jo-Jo was dead. When the horse ambulance arrived, I told them to take him to the hospital for a postmortem, although it was scarcely necessary.

Jo-Jo's rider said quietly to me, "Please save me some of his mane."

One thing especially impressed me about the police chargers. They are not toys. They are performing an important function and I think they realize it. There is a special bond between them and their riders that I have never seen anywhere else. I think the same bond must have existed between the old-time cavalryman and his mount. I remember reading that when the remnants of the Light Brigade rode back through the Valley of Death, one of the Russian batteries was still firing and men and horses were still falling. Many of the men refused to leave their dead or dying horses and sat crying beside them. I also recall a story told of a knight in the Middle Ages who remarked that he was eager to die and go to Heaven. When asked why, he replied simply, "Because I will meet Roland, my old warhorse, there."

IO

DISASTERS

I AM OFTEN ASKED, "WHAT WAS YOUR WORST DAY?" I CAN AN-
swer that with confidence: it was the day of the fire. Except for a
disaster involving human beings, I can't think of anything as
terrible as a fire in a stable full of livestock. It is my greatest
dread. If there is a word that means the opposite of a pyro-
maniac, that's me. I have such a horror of fire that I can't understand how firemen can go to them day after day without losing
their minds. Thank God they can, but I know it would kill me. I
have seen two barn fires involving horses and they were unbe-
lievably terrible.

The fire occurred at the Maui Meadows Breeding Farm, owned
by General and Mrs. Charles Lyman—renowned horse people—
where I was the farm veterinarian responsible for many areas.
Some mares resist being bred, some stallions are reluctant to
breed; then it's up to the veterinarian to try to overcome the difficulty. Even in cases where the animals are willing, the veterinarian should be present to check out the stallion's condition first and
make sure there is no infection he can transmit to the mare, and
also to prepare the mare and make sure she is at the period when
she is most likely to conceive. Then, after the breeding is over,
the veterinarian most often will take a sample of the stallion's
semen to ensure that it has the correct sperm count, that the
sperm is active, and that he has in fact ejaculated. As a mare has

an eleven-month gestation period, that's a long time to wait if there are no results. Equine veterinarians can now certify pregnancy after the covering so nothing is left to chance.

At the Maui Meadows farms, the leading thoroughred breeding farm in Pennsylvania, there was a fine gray stallion who had distinguished himself on the racetrack. Mr. Lyman now wanted him to stand at stud. There was only one problem. The stallion, although perfect in all other respects, refused to cover a mare. With the help of General Lyman's son Charles, who manages the farm, I was finally able to get him to mount the right mare and breed her, although it took us a week of hard, discouraging work. Once the stallion got the idea, there was no more trouble and we had every reason to believe that he would make a first-rate stud. I checked his spermatozoa with a microscope and they were perfect. Everyone was delighted with the results and I went home well satisfied. The stallion was not only a beautiful animal but remarkably gentle and I was personally fond of him. If I hadn't been able to get him to cover the mare, he would have been gelded and that would have been a disaster as he had magnificent bloodlines. So I was feeling proud of myself and had a special feeling toward the stud as one does toward any difficult animal or child that you have successfully brought around.

I remember it was on a Saturday evening. The next morning was a beautiful day. As it was Sunday, I determined to take some time off for myself, a decision I can seldom make. I was going to take a walk, work in the garden, relax, and do only the most important of my standard rounds.

At ten-thirty, I was just finishing breakfast and sipping a second cup of coffee when the telephone rang. I sighed and answered it, prepared for a routine call. It was a man, screaming, mad with hysteria. He shouted: "The barn's on fire! Come at once!" and hung up. He did not identify himself but I recognized the voice of the barn manager from the Maui Meadows farm in spite of the shrill, distorted tones.

I ran for the car. The barn was a magnificent old structure nearly a hundred years old—but I could not believe that the horses hadn't already been gotten out. There was a large and capable staff of grooms and stablemen. At night some of the horses might have been trapped, but it had been broad daylight for several hours, so the stable must have been full of people who would get the stock out at the first sign of trouble. Even so, I drove like crazy for the farm.

I was still 2 miles away when I saw the smoke rising like a giant black tree over the flat farmlands. I realized then for the first time that the whole barn must have gone up. How could it have happened? Some of the horses must have been trapped. I kept thinking, "Which ones?" and "How many?" Surely not my gray stallion. He was one of the most valuable animals. They'd have gotten him out first of all. I was so fearful that my knees felt weak.

When I was a mile away, the road was blocked with sightseers' cars, people who had seen the smoke and come to watch the fire. Why anyone would be attracted by a fire is a mystery to me. What is infinitely worse is that such people clog the highways, making it difficult for the fire engines, police cars, and ambulances to reach the site of the disaster. I tried to force my way through, leaning out of the window and shouting: "I'm a veterinarian—I have to get through! Maybe I can save some of the stock!" A few people grudgingly let me past but many refused to move. At last the police heard me and cleared a lane through which I drove, weaving around the cars.

Then I came to where the fire engines were parked. They were all over the place and the ground was a tangle of hoses like giant spaghetti. Ahead I could see a great mass of blood-red flames belching out black fountains of smoke that reached to the sky, all that was left of the beautiful barn. The smoke rolled up in billows like surf. Here not even the police could help me, yet I could not go on foot; I needed the medicines and instruments in my car. Somewhere in the fields were the horses, probably badly burned. I had to get through.

I saw some people standing by the engines and called out to them: "I'm a veterinarian! Please help me get through to where the horses are."

The crowd looked at me as though I were crazy. "There's no way you can get through. The road's blocked."

I pointed to the post-and-rail fence around the pasture. "Tear that down and I'll drive over the fields."

They hesitated, exchanged looks, then went for the fence. I

187

would like to have shot some of the gawkers who had blocked the road behind me, but this group responded magnificently. They lifted out the rails and even worked the posts loose and dragged them from the ground to clear a way. I shouted my thanks as I bounced over the fields. The heat from the burning barn was now so intense I had to circle it. Sparks and burning debris were falling all around me. Still, I could see no signs of horses or men.

Then came the most horrible sight I have ever witnessed: a horse running across the field on fire. His whole body was one big torch and he was screaming as he ran. It was the gray stallion that I had left only a few hours before. The farm manager and two other men were chasing him but there seemed no chance of their catching the desperate animal. I saw him vanish over a little hill, still burning as though he had been soaked in gasoline and still giving those hideous screams.

Finally I reached a place where the stable staff had managed to round up a pitiful few of the horses. Nearly all were badly burned. I began at once to put packs of sodium bicarbonate on their sores and inject them with painkillers. I also got out all my intravenous bottles and needles. While I was working, the men brought in the gray stallion. By some miracle, they had managed to corner him. He was so badly burned I despaired of saving him, but amazingly he survived, although he was so scarred that he could never be used as a stud. Ironically, the scars had nothing to do with his ability to father excellent foals, but people were turned off by his appearance.

Seventeen horses died in that fire, eleven colts and six fillies. All yearlings, all prime stock. The Lyman farm specialized in collecting animals that had rare and special bloodlines, many of which had taken years to develop. A number of the animals that died were the last of lines that could never be replaced. Simply by looking at the bodies you could tell instantly from which direction the fire had spread, for the horses had died in their stalls crowded in the corner furthest from the flames. All had their legs burned off, I suppose because the bedding in the stalls was inflammable. I had to identify each animal and sign a death certificate for the insurance company, a horrible task. Then I had to stand by while bulldozers dug the graves, which by law had to be at least 10 feet deep. Each body as it was dumped in reminded me of the times I had treated that animal, played with it, and looked forward to its future. Ever since then, if I see someone so much as smoking in a barn I go into a rage.

One of the stablemen had been mucking out a stall when the furnace exploded. What caused the explosion no one knows, but it went off like a bomb. The man saw a ball of fire come rolling down the aisle between the stalls. He barely managed to escape with his own life. The whole structure immediately went up in flames. Men rushed through the smoke and fire to tear open stall doors from the outside, but the horses refused to come out although five steps would have saved them. As is well known, horses completely panic in a fire and refuse to leave what seems to them the safety of their familiar stalls. One man told me with tears in his eyes, "I was determined to save some of the stock. We went into the stalls in spite of the heat and smoke and tried to drag the horses out. We beat them, kicked them, put ropes around their necks and pulled. We couldn't budge them."

Horses are unpredictable. Most of them refused to leave their stalls, but Charles Lyman, Jr., did save a young mare named Gypsy. He ran down the aisle, pulled open the door of her stall, and shouted her name. He could see her cowering in a corner but she refused to move. He tried to pull her out but it was impossible. The stall was fast filling with smoke and he could no longer breathe, so he staggered out into the aisle and fought his way to the door. Here he stopped and more in an unthinking frenzy than with any hope of response he once again shouted: *"Gypsy!"* Suddenly through the dense smoke Gypsy appeared, trotting toward him. She followed him out like a dog. All the others in this section of the barn perished.

There were also a number of show ponies in the barn. All these were saved—by a child. General Lyman's granddaughter was sleeping when the cry of "Fire!" first went up. In her nightgown and bare feet she ran to the barn, opened the stall door, and led out the ponies, who followed her readily. As the last one left, the roof collapsed behind them.

Maui Meadows never completely recovered from the tragedy.

189

Although the valuable stock could not be fully replaced, these courageous horsepeople continued in the thoroughbred breeding business.

My second worst day was the result not of intense heat but cold. I survived that day because I was a good deal younger than I am now. Also, I was very lucky.

It had started snowing late that afternoon. At first the flakes were no bigger than a thumbnail, but soon they were the size of oak leaves. They came down so thick we could no longer see the big maples lining our drive only a few yards from the house. In case of an emergency, Norma and I shoveled out the drive. The snow filled it in again almost as fast as we could shovel. Our fence had 3 inches of snow on it and the soft flakes muffled all sounds, so I felt as though I was in a dead world. To make matters worse, a wind sprang up, swirling the snow into vast drifts. Some of these were over our heads.

When we could do no more, we returned to the house, shook off as much snow as we could, and changed our clothes. For once, the telephone didn't ring and thankfully I went to sleep.

At one in the morning the phone went off. "I've got a mare foaling," came a voice. "She's having a hard time. Can you come at once?"

I looked out the window. The snow was still coming down as though someone was dumping gigantic baskets of white feathers over the window. The man lived in Bryn Mawr, 20 miles away. At that time Bryn Mawr was country; big estates with some scattered farms. This man lived on one of the farms and had several brood mares. His barn was 3 miles from the main road but I remembered that he had a bulldozer. Of course, he would have bulldozed a path to the highway. The question was, could I reach the farm? Unless the road plows were out and had swept the main roads, I doubted if I could.

Dear Father was alive in those days. He handled my business affairs, which have always been a problem with me, and tried to handle me too, as best he could. The telephone had awakened him and when he saw me getting ready to go out, he announced determinedly, "I'm going with you."

He was just recovering from a coronary. "Please don't," I begged him. "There's nothing you can do, and if you have another attack, it could be serious."

"I am positively not going to allow you to go out alone on a night like this," Father retorted. When he spoke like that, I knew it was no good arguing with him.

I'd had the foresight to put chains on the car and we got out of the driveway without any trouble. Once we hit the highway, our difficulties began. The plows had not gone through, or at least not in our neighborhood. Throughout the evening there had been just enough traffic so I could drive in the ruts left by previous cars although it was maddeningly slow going.

We were two hours getting to Bryn Mawr and the farm. Then came another shock: the man had not cleared a path to his barn. It turned out that he had been so busy with the mare he had forgotten all about it and never considered how I would get to the stable over the snow-covered path. Luckily, the wind had swept across the open fields and blown much of the snow away so we were able to crawl along, expecting to be mired down at any moment.

Then we came to a double barrier about a mile from the barn. There was a drift higher than the car's hood, which extended like a wall as far as we could see in either direction. Not only that, but the weight of the snow had brought down a power line running from the main house to the stable and a tangle of wires lay embedded in the snow, some coils barely showing above the surface, others entirely buried.

I told Father, "I'll have to go on foot from here and carry whatever I can. You wait for me. Run the heater but leave one window open a crack in case of carbon monoxide."

"Don't worry about me," Father said calmly. "I'll be fine. I only wish I could help you carry something, but I know quite well I'd never make it through that drift."

We had some blankets and I made him as comfortable as I could in the back seat of the car. When I got out, I went over my knees in the snow and only just managed to wade to the back of the car and get out what equipment I thought I'd need. Then I started out for the barn.

I knew without trying that I couldn't possibly get through the drift; I'd have to go around it. It was impossible to avoid the wires. I went over them and between them. By some incredible chance, I did not touch any; why, I can't imagine, as I couldn't tell where most of them were. The drift seemed to stretch for miles and sometimes I was up to my waist in snow. Then I came on a little grove of pines. These had served as a windbreak and the snow was only a few inches deep here. By keeping to the grove, I was able to get around the drift and saw before me the lighted windows of the stable. It was all downhill.

When I staggered into the barn, a group of men were in the stall with the mare. One of them looked up and asked in astonishment, "How did you ever get here?"

"If you didn't expect me to get here, why did you send for me?" I demanded, understandably annoyed.

No one had an answer to that, so I examined the mare.

She was uncomfortable, intractable, and sweating freely, which usually means birth is imminent. As she was obviously in pain, I sedated her and scrubbed up in some hot water and soap the men brought me. Then I scrubbed the mare. She was straining to deliver the foal but nothing came.

"What's wrong, Doctor?" asked the owner.

"I'm not sure," I admitted. "I think the foal must be twisted in some way."

A foal should be born forefeet first, one foreleg extended and slightly preceding the other, with the nose between the legs. If any other parts appear first, the foal must be turned, which means there is a chance that both the foal and the mare will die. No room for error—nature leaves no extra space.

I reached inside the mare's body. Yes, I could feel the foal and it was alive. I soon located the trouble. The legs were twisted. I straightened them and the little animal slipped out. She was a nice little chestnut filly. Then I wiped the nostrils clean and set the little girl on her grasshopper legs. The afterbirth appeared scanty but that is often the case with a small foal. Yet the mare appeared uneasy, restless, and showed no interest in the foal, which is most unusual. Some mares have a postpartum cramp in an attempt to pass the afterbirth and I thought this was the trou-

192

ble. Then she broke into a sweat and dropped down, assuming the position for giving birth, which startled us all. I scrubbed up again, both myself and the mare.

I would have to examine her a second time. I did so and for a few seconds couldn't believe what my fingers told me was a fact. There was a second foal in her. Twins are almost unknown among horses; in all my experience I have only seen one other pair. But this foal had a sister or a brother. Unfortunately the second foal was badly twisted, a breech delivery. Taking the greatest pains not to let the sharp little hoofs tear the uterus, I gradually worked it into position. It was a long and delicate job but I had almost succeeded when a stableman rushed in. "Come quick, doc!" he shouted. "There's a mare in the far stall giving birth."

I might have known it. If a mare gives birth and there is another mare in the same barn near her time, she will try desperately to give birth also. I believe it is the odor that triggers the reaction.

"If I leave this mare now, you'll have a dead foal and a dead mare," I told the owner. "The other mare will just have to wait."

"She's having a lot of trouble," said the stableman doubtfully.

"Which ones do you want to save?" I asked the owner.

He hesitated a moment. "You keep on here. We'll do what we can for the other mare."

There was a strong temptation to hurry matters but that could be fatal. I forced myself to work slowly, not taking any chances, and tried to forget about the other mare. At last I was able to slide the foal out onto the straw. It was another chestnut filly, an identical twin to the first. In the rare cases when a mare does have twins, they are nearly always of different sizes, one much larger than the other. These two were exactly the same.

One of the grooms had stayed with me. "Clean out her nostrils, then rub her down and get her nursing," I told him urgently. Grabbing my bag, I ran down the aisle to the far stall. There was the mare, straining hard, with a group of men standing helplessly around her. I soon found out what the matter was: the foal was huge. By the time I got him out (it was a colt), the mother was so exhausted that she would have to have intravenous injections and supportive therapy. But the mother of the twins also needed help. I had only brought along enough drugs for one animal—I would have to go back to the car.

Daylight was just beginning to break. Although I had broken a trail through the snow and knew the way, this trip seemed harder than the first. I was worn out and my legs were so heavy I could barely force them through the snow. There was no use sending one of the men; he wouldn't have known what drugs to take from the car. I was also worried about Father, who was in no shape to sit in a drafty car stuck in a snowdrift. When I finally saw the car ahead of me and shouted, it was with infinite relief that I heard him answer.

"Are you all right?" I yelled.

"Never better. Did you deliver the foal?"

I explained what had happened, and climbing over the downed wires again, I got the drugs and instruments I needed. Poor Father gallantly offered to help me carry them, but it would have been suicide for him to have attempted the trip. Loaded down for the second time, I forced my way over the wires, around the drift, and through the grove. Thank heaven, it had stopped snowing. Back in the barn, I gave both animals I.V.'s and antibiotic injections. I also gave them stress injections. When I saw all three foals nursing and was sure the mares were out of danger, I made my third trip through the snow across the wires and fell into the car. Father drove me home. I don't remember getting into bed, and only woke up at eleven o'clock. I drove back to the stable to check on my patients, who were all doing well.

Afterwards, before starting out on my regular rounds, I stopped in at a diner for some coffee. A policeman I knew was there and we said hello.

"You won't believe this, Dr. Lose," he told me, "but the electric wires on the breeding farm near Bryn Mawr came down in the storm last night and some damned fool crawled across them to get to the stable. They're live wires. Why he wasn't killed, I'll never know. Can you imagine anyone being that dumb?"

"Well, it takes all kinds," I agreed.

The single colt grew up to distinguish himself on the racetrack. The twins unfortunately both had umbilical hernias and I had a hard time pulling one through as it had strangulated. Nevertheless, both recovered and became strong, healthy mares, although not good enough for the track. They were sold as saddle horses and led happy lives.

Both these mares were good mothers. When a mare rejects her foal, it can be a serious matter because of the vital importance of the first milk, which has a high antibody and laxative content. Once at Mr. Biddle's farm I was called in to handle one of the strangest cases of foal rejection I can remember.

I got a call to come to the Biddle stable "as quickly as possible," which I knew meant a fairly serious emergency as Mr. Biddle wasn't the nervous type. I was by myself that day and as I knew all the back roads in that part of the country where there wouldn't be any traffic, I made good time. Mr. Biddle had fifteen brood mares, all of which were in foal, running together in one of his big fields; but now they were all gathered together in the paddock of one of his stables. When I arrived, Mr. Biddle took me to a stall where a newborn foal stood swaying uncertainly on its long legs. The foal was all alone, pathetic and whinnying for its mother, bruised and weakening.

"Where's the mother?" I asked, anxious as always to get the foal nursing as quickly as possible.

"That's why I brought you over," replied Mr. Biddle. "We saw the mares in the field kicking and snapping at something, then throwing up their heads, galloping away, and coming back to attack again. One of the men went over to investigate and found this little foal lying on the grass. We can't see any sign of any of the mares having given birth, yet the foal must belong to one of them. None of the mares shows any interest in it."

This was a new one to me. I gave the mares a quick check, examining the vulvas and checking to see if the mammary glands had milk. I could find nothing. Often young mares show very little sign of having delivered and the milk does not come in until the foal starts nursing. Yet there had to be some indications if I could only recognize them. Some maiden mares deliver (especially in an open field), get up, and walk away—perhaps thinking the pain was a colic attack, not looking back, and most important not smelling the "telltale odor" that usually signals the brain.

I began again. This time, I found some extremely slight indications in the vulva and udder of a maiden mare. We put her in the stall with the foal and she at once attacked it. Neglect I had seen, especially with mares who had never had a foal before and did not realize what the strange little creature was, but never aggression. There were no signs of the placenta, which when expelled in a field is readily destroyed by dogs, cats, and large birds.

"Do you want a nose twitch?" asked Mr. Biddle.

"I'd better tranquilize her first," I told him. As soon as the mare was under sedation, she grew more quiet and I brought the foal over to her. In spite of the tranquilizer, she turned on him.

"I guess we'll need that nose twitch after all," I admitted. With a groom holding her and heavily tranquilized, the mare had no choice but to allow the foal to nurse on the scantly developed udder and small teats. I stayed there until after the tranquilizer wore off and the groom released the nose twitch but still held the mare by a lead shank to her halter. While we all watched, hardly daring to breathe, the mare turned and nuzzled the little foal. Then she licked him. It was going to be all right. The mare turned out to be an almost overly protective mother, for she was apt to attack anyone going into the stall in an effort to protect the foal. We never did find the afterbirth!

I suggested that the rest of the mares be kept in individual stalls until they had given birth. I have never seen horses attack a newborn foal as these did, nor a mother so totally indifferent to her offspring. It is just another mystery of the horse world I can't explain.

Often in my practice I have had to make hard decisions. Some of these decisions have caused my clients bitter disappointments. There are veterinarians who will refuse to tell a client something that might antagonize him or her. This is partly because they want to avoid trouble and partly because it almost surely means losing the client. In the past, I have regarded veterinarians who are afraid to face up to the truth as being cowardly, but perhaps I am being unfair. After all, any veterinarian can be wrong, and perhaps these shillyshalliers are merely giving an animal the benefit of the doubt. I remember especially two cases where I was absolutely positive of my diagnosis. In one case, I stuck to my belief and may well have saved a child's life; in the other, I was overruled and it turned out that I was wrong.

A wealthy couple had a fifteen-year-old daughter who was "horse-crazy," as many young girls are. I had watched her riding at pony shows and she took her hobby very seriously and worked hard at it. Her parents were devoted to her but tried not to spoil her, in general succeeding. She could have virtually anything she wanted—once her parents were convinced that she'd really earned it. The girl was especially fond of show jumping and wanted a good young show hunter. At one show she had fallen in love with a magnificent chestnut standing 17 hands that had come off with all the ribbons. He was a champion and had won at a number of major shows. The girl had hopefully asked if he was for sale and the owner said yes—for $50,000. The girl turned away with a sigh but her father had heard.

A few days later he called me. "Dr. Lose, I'm going to get that hunter for my girl," he told me. "That is, of course, if the horse is warranted sound. Will you come up to the stable in Connecticut and vet the horse for me? It's just a formality as he's a champion and has been winning wherever he's shown, but I want to be sure. My wife and daughter will be going with me, only don't tell my daughter anything. I want it to be a surprise for her."

"I won't, but don't you tell the owner that we're coming," I warned. "I don't know anything about the man but it's easy with drugs and tricks of one kind and another to cover up faults in a horse if you know he's going to be vetted. Let's just drop in on him."

"Right," agreed my friend. "We'll leave tomorrow at ten."

I have to drive so much that I dread long drives, only this one was a pleasure. We went up in a big, comfortable car with special seats and for once I could really relax. There was a large trunk where I stored all the veterinary equipment I thought I'd need, even including a portable X-ray outfit. After all, $50,000 is a great deal of money and I didn't want there to be any mistakes. I forget now what story they'd told the girl; at any rate she chatted away happily and the drive seemed short.

At the stable, the owner wasn't present but his manager was. I took a dislike to the man; he was the high-powered type who wants to rush you off your feet. The girl recognized the horse instantly and went half-crazy with excitement. He was indeed a magnificent animal: I believe his conformation was the best I've ever seen. As for his record, it spoke for itself.

"Let's close the deal now," suggested the manager. "The little lady and the horse have fallen in love with each other. Why go to a lot of unnecessary trouble? You can see for yourselves that the horse is perfect."

The girl's parents were willing to forego the examination. However, having brought me all the way to Connecticut, they decided I'd better go through the formality of making a check-up. As the horse was led out of the stall, it seemed to me he had a curious look in his eyes, but I put that down to my imagination. A professional rider mounted him and he was put through his paces and over some jumps. Perfect. I X-rayed him. Perfect. I examined his legs, listened to his heart, checked his lungs. Perfect.

"Now take him back to the barn and turn off the lights," I told the manager, although again the horse was obviously sound and this was simply a formality.

For the first time the manager looked disturbed. "Aren't you making a big fuss over nothing?" he asked. "I suppose you have to show that you're earning your fee, but enough is enough."

I remembered the strange expression in the horse's eyes. "I'm afraid that I'll have to insist."

In the darkened barn, I checked the horse's eyes with an ophthalmoscope: he had only 30 percent vision. The retinal vessels were hazy, imperfect, and the lens capsule contained precipitates.

The girl was happily dancing around, announcing her plans for showing her wonderful new horse. Her parents were smiling at her delight. Her father asked confidently, "Well, everything all right, Dr. Lose?"

I couldn't bear to tell them. All I could say was, "Turn on the lights." The manager took one look at my face, swore, and stamped out of the barn. There was a groom standing there and I asked him quietly, "How long has he been like this? It looks like a systemic disease to me and it will gradually get worse."

The groom hesitated, then said, "He's had it for years, but with a really good rider who knows him, it doesn't make much difference. You just have to be extra careful how you bring him into the ring, clue him when to jump, and make sure he knows exactly where the jump is."

I walked out of the barn in silence. The girl was still jumping with delight and kept repeating, "I love that horse so much. We'll have such good times together. When can we van him home?" Her mother said delightedly, "I've never seen her so happy about anything. I was so worried the horse might have been sold. It would have broken her heart."

I would have given a great deal not to tell them the truth. I thought desperately of some way to avoid the issue. If there had been any operation that could have helped the animal, or if the girl had only wanted him as a saddle horse to hack around on, I would have been sorely tempted to keep quiet. I knew I was going to hurt the girl cruelly and gravely disappoint her parents, but there was nothing I could do. Finally I blurted out, "That horse is going blind. In fact, he's half-blind already. It would be a terrible mistake to buy him for anyone, especially a child."

The little girl stared at me as though I had slashed her across the face with a whip. Then she broke into hysterical sobs that were frightening. Her mother led her to the car while her father stared at me and asked, "Are you sure?"

"Positive."

"Then how is the animal winning ribbons?"

"He's always ridden by a professional who knows about his vision problem. A rider like that can put the horse in exactly the right position to take off, signal him with reins and knees how to jump, and make sure he isn't put into any event where there are jumps he wouldn't be accustomed to take. A really good rider could probably take a blind horse around the ring like that. It's dangerous, but they're paid to take risks. Your daughter hasn't the skill for anything like that and she isn't being paid to risk her life."

The man looked at me. For an instant, I thought he was going to call me a liar. Then he turned away and we went back to the car, where the disappointed child was crying in her mother's arms. The mother looked at me as though I were a murderess—and I felt like one.

The girl cried all the way back to Pennsylvania. Her mother kept saying, "We'll get you another horse," to which the tearful girl always replied, "I don't want another horse. I'll never ride again." Neither of the parents spoke to me. It was the longest drive I can remember. I unpacked my heavy X-ray equipment and other gear, transferred them to my car without anyone offering to help, and drove home. I arrived shortly after midnight, feeling as though I'd had one of the most tiring days of my life.

Two months later, I ran into the father at a horse show. He remarked casually, "Do you remember that horse in Connecticut you said was partly blind?"

I looked at him in considerable surprise. "Yes, of course, I remember him well."

"Our daughter was so broken up about not getting him that I took the family to Florida for a vacation. We went to a horse show there and damned if there wasn't the very horse we'd nearly bought in Connecticut. His owner had flown him down for the Florida show circuit and we saw him jump. The first jump on the course was an easy one; a brush jump only about two and a half feet high. His rider put him at it, but instead of jumping he went right into it. Fell and rolled on his rider. They had to destroy the horse immediately and they took the rider off in an ambulance." He looked at me oddly. "You know, Doctor, you were right after all about that horse not being able to see."

I stared at him. "You mean you thought I didn't know what I was talking about?"

He looked away. "Well, I didn't say that exactly. Only it's possible—anyone can be wrong."

I felt a hollow sensation in my stomach. Although, thank heaven, this couple had followed my advice, they had clearly considered me incompetent. It was a bad blow to my pride.

However, he was right. I can be wrong, I'm sorry to say—or in this particular case, perhaps I should say, "I'm glad to say." In 1976 I was called in to examine the horses of the great wagon train encamped at Valley Forge Park. As part of the Bicentennial celebration, people were invited to visit Philadelphia from all parts of the country in horse-drawn wagons. I couldn't believe how many came; there were scores of them, some from as far as California. Almost certainly no such exhibition can ever be made again, for horse-drawn wagons and draft horses are fast vanishing.

I drove to the park along Yellow Springs Road, still lined by big old estates, some dating back to Colonial days, and across Knox Covered Bridge and along Valley Creek toward Washington's headquarters, which is still preserved in exactly the same condition as it was during that fearful winter, "the low point of the Revolution," when a little band of determined men made their last stand among these hills. I passed what is left of the original forge in the valley that gave the district its name, drove along the ridge where replicas of the log cabins used by the troops stand, and alongside the earthern gun emplacements with their long lines of cannons. Many of the pre-Revolutionary buildings are still standing and still occupied: the bakehouse that provided bread for the troops; the Great Valley Mill, where the flour was ground and which until a few years ago was still operating; the powder house where the guns were repaired; Lafayette's headquarters; and the lovely King of Prussia Inn, now isolated by the new expressway but once a delightful spot where the foxhounds met regularly and delicious meals were served as they had been ever since 1709.

It was one of the hottest Julys on record. I remember it was 95 degrees with not a cloud in the sky. Everywhere were campers, trailers, tents, and wagons, plus thousands of sightseers' cars blocking the highway. There was no way to get past them, so I was obliged to drive over the grass, a fearful crime in the eyes of the park authorities, but the police recognized my car and waved me through. The wagons were of all shapes and sizes and seemed in remarkably good condition considering the hundreds—in some cases, thousands—of miles they had traveled. There were lots of mules and donkeys as well as the draft horses. All had borium on their shoes to give them better footing on the paved roads, a wise precaution. One especially big wagon had an eight-mule team hitch, the largest I'd ever seen.

I introduced myself and was shown around. The people were real old American stock, polite, rugged, independent, rather taciturn, and obviously skillful at handling both their equipment and stock. One man was over eighty. There were surprisingly few saddle or harness sores. What injuries there were seemed mainly to be hurt coronary bands and minor abrasions on the horses' legs. Naturally the horses had lost some weight on the long trip but were rapidly gaining it back. I was especially impressed by the saddle horses, which had remarkably strong backs. Clearly they were bred for real work rather than for recreation as in the East.

An elderly couple approached me and the man said courteously, "Doctor, I'd be grateful if you'd look at our mare. She had a foal a couple of hours ago."

I stared at him. "Where did you come from?"

"Alaska." He spoke as though it were the next county.

"You mean you brought a mare in foal nearly four thousand miles on foot?"

"That's right. My son was riding her." He indicated a well-set-up young man who smiled and bobbed his head to me.

I took a long breath. "Is the foal alive?"

The man looked surprised. "Surely. Doing well."

All I could think was that people and horses are a sturdy breed in Alaska. I checked the mare. She was in excellent shape, although rather thin. Just to be sure, I gave her some antibiotics to prevent infection and an intravenous injection to build up her strength. Then I asked to see the foal.

I got a shock. The foal, only a few hours old, was out in the roasting sun. She was weak, undernourished, and panting from the cruel heat. Her umbilical cord was dragging on the ground, swollen and covered with filth. The little creature was surrounded by a curious crowd who apparently had never seen a foal before, all shouting and taking pictures, some of them pulling her about as though she were a toy.

"She's the hit of the whole wagon train," the man told me proudly. "The newspapers have played her up big. Yes, sir, you could say she's the star attraction."

"She won't be for very long at this rate," I told him. "If you leave her out in the sun like this, she'll be dead in a few hours."

My first concern was the contaminated and perhaps infected umbilical cord. I had the man and his wife hold the pathetic little creature while I amputated the cord and cleaned the incision with iodine. Then I injected her with antitoxin. All this had to be done in the open, on filthy, dusty ground, in the incredible heat of the midday sun with no shade.

"Now, we'll have to get her where she can rest and out of the sun," I explained. "I know a man not far from here with a stable and I'm sure he'll let her stay there with the mare. It will be comparatively cool—it's a big, airy barn—and she'll be out of the sun and away from these people. I'll carry her and you follow with the mare."

The man shook his head. "I can't do that, lady. Like I said, she's the big hit of the show. Everybody's coming around to ask about her. In a stable, no one can see her."

"She'll be dead by evening if you leave her here," I told him. "I'll pledge my professional reputation on it."

The mother broke in. "All our stock's plenty tough. She'll be all right."

I argued and argued. I even thought of threatening them with the SPCA. Nothing produced any impression. Other members of the wagon train began to gather around us in a menacing way. They, too, recognized the foal as a big attraction and didn't want it moved. All the members of the train stuck together; they had traveled far and felt like a family standing up against "easterners." As the foal was practically dead already, I finally decided there was no use making an issue out of the sad business. When I left I said, "At least put her under a tree where she can have some shade and some cool grass to lie on."

"Can't do it," explained the man. "People can take her picture better out here in the sun."

Yet these people clearly loved their horses and took good care of them. It was incredible.

I returned the next day to continue my vetting and treating of the stock. I glanced around to see what they had done with the corpse of the foal, which by now must surely be dead; there had been scarcely any life in it the previous afternoon. To my astonishment, there was the little animal, still out in the broiling sun and even looking a little stronger. I couldn't understand it. I gave the foal another injection and again pleaded with the owners if they wouldn't put it in the stable—which was only a quarter of a mile away—at least to provide it with some shade. Again they refused.

That autumn, the wagon train broke up and the various units started for home. Among them were the foal's owners. By then, the foal was in fine shape: healthy, playful, and fat. She trotted off after the mare, fully prepared for the 4,000-mile trip, and I'm willing to bet she made it. When the woman said, "Our stock's plenty tough," she wasn't exaggerating. I'd have bet $1,000 against a plugged nickel that that foal couldn't possibly have survived those first days of exposure. I am happy to say that I was wrong.

As my practice expanded, I was able to keep going only with the help of my family. Actually, "my practice" was a family affair rather than a one-person affair. I'd like to tell one story to show what I mean.

I've never had a very good head for business and also I simply don't have the time. My father always handled my business affairs for me. I have trouble keeping up with the latest medical research since I don't have the time to read the current papers put out from the research centers. Of late, there has been a great improvement here. The papers are put on cassette tapes, which I can play while driving from one farm to another. That has made a big difference. When Father died, Mother and Norma took over the bookkeeping, for which I thank heaven and them. Unhappily, none of us has Father's business background and knowledge of affairs.

Norma handles the phone calls. I can't tell you how important this is. I've heard it said, "The person on the phone can make or break a veterinarian," and I believe it. No matter how tired Norma is or what hour she has been gotten out of bed, she is always eager and interested. Nothing so infuriates an anxious owner as if the veterinarian's answering service sounds rude or even indifferent. He's worried sick and he expects you to be. Then too there's the problem of emergency calls. To the owner, his call is an emergency even though it may be a minor matter. If a police horse has been hit by a truck or a mare is dying while foaling, I must go there first. However, I always make it a point to arrange with some other veterinarian to take emergency calls if I'm away. Norma must decide how important is the call and, if I can't make it, who can best handle the case. But I think her hardest job is explaining why I am so often late. I'll allow, say, twenty minutes for a call. When I'm finished, my client often says, "Now as long as you're here, I wish you'd look at. . . ." That may mean another hour. Meanwhile, people expecting me are calling Norma and she has to explain why I'm delayed.

Mother spells me at driving. Often I have what we call an "elastic" day, meaning unexpected calls and long, extra hours. On occasion, I've gone for forty-eight hours without a break. I couldn't do it alone. Mother does the driving and I'm fortunate enough to be able to sleep sitting up in the car beside her. Father had the same faculty. It comes in very handy.

Margaret, my niece, began helping me when she was ten years old. Now that she's twenty-two, she has become my main assistant. I've asked her if she would like to be a veterinarian and her reply is, "Why spend eight years reading books when I can learn on the job?" Of course, without a veterinarian's license she can never practice on her own, but without her, I'd have to curtail my work drastically. She knows where all the drugs and instruments are and assists at surgery. If I'm miles away and find that I need something, I can call home on the car radio. Margaret will prepare whatever it is I want, then she and Mother will meet me at some agreed-on point so I can keep going.

I remember one of these "elastic" days in particular. I had been going steadily since five in the morning and I got home at ten that night. I took a hot bath, and was climbing into bed when the telephone rang. It was the Lyman stables. A horse had gotten lacerated, was bleeding badly, and needed instant attention.

I was too exhausted to drive, so Mother took the wheel while Margaret went along to help. She is an expert anesthetist and it sounded as though she might be needed. It was a half hour's drive to Lyman's and I found a thoroughbred seriously·cut up. He had to be sutured carefully so as not to leave any disfiguring scars. It was two in the morning before I finished.

As we went back to the car, I began to feel sick. I'm generally a healthy person but the day before I'd made the mistake of stopping at a diner for a sandwich because I didn't have time to eat anywhere else. Norma usually packs a lunch for me so I can eat while driving, but this time we hadn't anticipated the rush of calls that turned up so she hadn't bothered. The sandwich had been bad and I should never have eaten it, only I was hungry and in a hurry. Now I was paying for it.

"I'm going to be sick," I told Mother, as I crawled into the car. "Let's get home as quickly as possible."

There was still a delay. Margaret had to clean, pack, and arrange all the instruments I'd used. We have a cast-iron rule about this. I have learned from bitter experience that if the instruments are simply tossed into the car to be cleaned and properly packed later, we invariably get an emergency call. That means when we arrive on the case, everything has to be sorted out and cold-sterilized. Where time is vital, such a delay can be fatal to the patient. Thank heaven I had Margaret there to do the long, tedious job as I certainly wasn't up to it. I lay in my seat, twisted by stomach cramps, until Margaret had finished. In half an hour, I'd be home in bed.

Then the radio crackled. It was Norma. Even before I could understand what she was saying, I knew by her tone that it was another emergency. "There's a sick mare at the Pancoast stables," she told us anxiously. "She's in foal and was just shipped up from Florida. It's a bad case of bloat-colic. Her temperature is a hundred and three. They're afraid they'll lose both the foal and the mare, so hurry."

The Pancoast stable was an hour away. Mother picked up the receiver. "Phyllis is sick. Tell them to get someone else." Back came Norma's voice: "I could tell Phyllis wasn't well when she left for the Lymans'. I've been trying to find another veterinarian. No one will answer at this hour. The Pancoasts are counting on her."

I'd been the Pancoasts' veterinarian for fifteen years. They had a racing stable and breeding farm and it had been one of my first really important assignments. They had never used another veterinarian in all that time and I couldn't let them down. I took the mike from Mother. "Tell them we'll be there as soon as possible."

Mother did not say anything but drove as fast as she could. I was feeling sicker every minute. Several times I thought I couldn't make it and we'd have to give up, but each time the thought of the mare kept me going. At last we reached the Pancoast stables and I fell out of the car. Two men were walking a big brood mare around in circles. There was no doubt that she was sick—even sicker than I was. She had broken out into a heavy perspiration and was enormously bloated. One good thing, I had a preparation that is a sovereign cure for colic. I turned to Margaret. She was standing behind me with everything ready: tube, colic medicine, antacid sedation, and mineral oil. I injected intravenously to quiet her and ease the pain. Then we tubed her and pumped the mixture down into her stomach. Two hours later, she was all right and we could start home. Dawn was just coming up when we reached Berwyn. I barely made it to bed. Shortly afterwards, I had to start out on my regular rounds.

II

MY OWN HOSPITAL

ALMOST FROM THE TIME THAT I FIRST STARTED PRACTICING, I sorely missed not having my own veterinary hospital. There are two excellent animal hospitals in the general Philadelphia area, but both insist that any animal entering them is to be treated only by their own staff. That, of course, meant that I lost all contact with the patient. There was no chance for extended observation, no opportunity for intensive care, and I could not perform any surgery. Under these circumstances, I felt like only half a doctor.

Neither could I conduct any experiments. My three great interests were orthopedic and hoof diseases, and working with brood mares and foals. Horses often go lame; twenty years ago, it was pretty much taken for granted that they had to be destroyed. After numerous dissections, I noticed that the trouble observed in the malformed foot was often due to the contraction of the flexor tendon in the foreleg of young horses. In the same sheath as the deep flexor tendon is a check ligament that is attached to the cannon bone. When the check ligament is too short, there is a disparity between the bone growth and the tendon. As a result, the horse is "standing on tiptoe," as it were. Not only is this very painful but the end of the toe tends to open, permitting bacteria to enter and putting additional pressure on the coronary band. To allow the horse to put his foot flat on the ground, the check ligament would have to be lengthened.

This was my theory, shared with a few other individuals. Testing it was something else again. The condition could be corrected in part by using casts, stretching the tendon, and other methods. None were satisfactory, but without my own hospital I was unable to experiment.

I also ran into frequent problems with brood mares and their foals. Occasionally a foal would retain the meconium (the first intestinal discharge of a newborn animal). This sometimes required surgery to correct. Other foals would develop hernias; often these could be reduced temporarily by manual manipulation, but when they were caused by development of adhesions or by an entrapped loop of intestine, then surgery was necessary. Again, a foal may rupture its bladder at birth, especially if the mare becomes startled and jumps to her feet prematurely, giving a sharp jerk on the intact umbilical cord. Then there are the leg problems, such as an extreme case of "knock knees," when the forelegs are literally pressed together and can be straightened only by a surgical process; then there is the opposite, leaving the horse "bow-legged."*

Either these often delicate operations had to be performed in an unsanitary stall without any proper facilities or the animal had to be sent to a hospital and treated by another veterinarian, who often had very different ideas about how to deal with these problems. Further, both these hospitals were attached to veterinary schools where students were allowed to work on the patients. Naturally I realize that students must be trained, just as I was, but sometimes this puts quite a strain on the animal. But worst of all I was never able to test any of my theories on how to correct these conditions as I was not on the staff of either hospital.

So for years I dreamed about having my own hospital. I made sketches of it. I read everything I could find on the subject of animal hospitals, and even managed to take off enough time to travel around the country and inspect all the leading equine hospitals. I found very few good ones. Yet building my own seemed hopeless. I had no credit rating and my own expenses were so

---

* These problems and many more are discussed fully in my book *Blessed Are the Brood Mares* (New York: Macmillan Publishing Co., Inc., 1978).

great that I was barely able to keep solvent no matter how my practice expanded.

Finally, in 1970, with the help of Malcolm Meyer at the Berwyn Bank and some friends, plus the extra income I was getting from the mounted police, the miracle happened: I could build my hospital. To comply with the zoning restrictions, mother generously gave me 10 acres; enough not only for my hospital but also for several paddocks surrounded by post-and-board fencing, where recuperating patients could gallop and play.

I already had an old carriage house, dating back to Colonial times, which contained five box stalls and four "straight" stalls. This I used for animals who were not seriously ill and had no contagious diseases. Near it was a cottage that we rented out. To comply with the zoning laws, all buildings had to be clustered together with several acres of open land around them. According to my plans, the hospital would cover approximately 1 acre and so it would have to be built next to the carriage house and cottage.

I did my best to have the hospital resemble the older buildings. It was made of cement blocks, painted white, with a roof of black asbestos shingles to match the stone and dark wood shingles of the other structures. Near it is a magnificent sugar maple that I think must be at least two hundred years old, which I protected by a concrete wall and which provides good shade. Many of the clinics I had seen were models of human hospitals with only a few modifications. As this was to be solely an equine hospital, without any other animal patients, I had to have virtually everything specially designed. I insisted on complete temperature control, including total air conditioning, with each area controlled by its own thermostat. Inside, the cement blocks are covered with epoxy glaze tile so the walls could be easily cleaned. All the electrical outlets are capped, waterproofed, and made of shock-resistant stainless steel. The surgical faucets were designed by me and custom-built.

A patient first enters the ward. There are fifteen box stalls, each with heavy-duty metal counterbalanced doors I designed myself. Each unit has its own individual lighting, air conditioning, and heat control. The stalls are equipped with Nelson self-waterers and there are individual haydrops and grain dispensers that connect to the loft above. We keep at least six hundred bales of hay in the loft at all times, brought from our farm upstate. Stainless steel doors that can be controlled electrically to roll up or down connect the ward to the outside and also lead into the clinic. At the other end is a fully equipped blacksmith's shop, with a forge, two anvils, and all the necessary tools.

I decided that the best flooring throughout this area would be Dynafarm, which I had to import from Germany. It is impervious to acids, heat, and corrosives, and does not mark from borium shoes (shoes treated in a special way to give a horse better footing on smooth surfaces). Dynafarm also has a special resilient base that adds to a horse's comfort.

A horse requiring surgery is first given a sedative in the ward, then led into the main clinic. The clinic is by far the largest room in the hospital, measuring 150 by 50 feet. I wanted it this big so I could have a horse trotted up and down to study his action if necessary. At the far end is a structure we call the orthopedic stall. This is very solidly built, with wooden bars; a horse can be led in and fastened securely in place so he cannot move. Slings can even be lowered from the top of the stall so the animal can be lifted off his feet. I use it for minor surgery, standing procedures, examinations, and so on.

For major surgery, the animal is put into the part of the clinic known as the induction area. The floor here is coated with 6 inches of foam rubber covered with heavy duck cloth that can be washed. The walls are also padded. Here the horse is given an injection that anesthetizes him, so that he slides down onto a mat. The anesthetist intubates with a long rubber tube placed into the trachea and then begins the maintenance anesthetic in the form of gas—usually halothane. If the operation is to be a long one, I.V. supportive fluids are routinely used.

Set in the floor is a "lift"—a movable section of flooring the size of a horse. A wheeled table is rolled over the lift, and by pressing a button, the lift can be made to sink down until the top of the table is flush with the floor. An inflatable mat filled with air, with the horse lying on it, is pulled over the table. The lift then rises until the table can be rolled off it. Then the table is rolled across the clinic to the far end where a stainless-steel door rises electrically to give admission to the surgical prep room, where the horse is recleaned, reprepared, and then rough draped for surgery. This area, together with the surgery, has its own generator in case of a power failure in the main unit. The sinks are of stainless steel; the faucets can be knee-operated, and the soap dispenser foot-operated, for the use of the surgeon and his assistants. Here the floor is of Mypolam, a special conductive surgical flooring that has metal filing embedded in it so there is no danger of electric shock to patient or surgeon from static electricity.

In the surgery the light is Skytron, imported from Japan; the room is equipped with fourteen sealed-beam lights in the large unit and five in the satellite unit. No matter where I stand, this light gives a shadow-free, nondistorted view of the surgical field. The table is so adjusted that by a touch of the finger it swings into any position. There is a large observation window between the reception room (which also includes my office) and the surgery, for students, owners, and trainers, so they can watch operations without making it necessary for them actually to enter the surgery.

After the operation the horse is wheeled back into the clinic and, through another stainless-steel door, into the recovery room. This has padded walls and a padded floor; there is a special air mattress onto which the horse is lowered, and the room has a closed-circuit television so the patient can be kept under observation at all times. In addition, two windows of shatter-proof glass are set at different levels for direct observation.

The pharmacy also connects with the clinic. This room measures roughly 45 by 30 feet. The walls are lined with built-in cabinets and counters, and there is a stainless-steel opening into the clinic through which medications and equipment can be passed. When not in use, this opening can be sealed off from the clinic by a steel sliding door. In the pharmacy are two autoclaves (units of steam under pressure for sterilizing instruments). These are based on designs used in ordinary hospitals but had to be custom-built as the equine instruments are larger. There is a darkroom where X-rays are developed by the Picker developer, which can produce a dry radiograph in ninety seconds. In addition, there are several smaller rooms, such as the dressing room where the staff change; nearby is a commercial-sized washer and dryer. The garage, which houses the mobile clinic as well as two ordinary cars, connects with the pharmacy.

As far as I know, this is the most fully equipped privately owned equine hospital in the world. Certainly I know of none in the United States to equal it, and visitors from Europe have assured me that they have never seen any in their own countries so complete. I now spend more time in my hospital than I do on the road. I am proud to say that it was awarded national honors for design and organization. Today the hospital and equipment is valued at $1.5 million.

In addition to Norma and my niece Margaret, my staff consisted of Nancy Fisher, a registered nurse who assists me in surgical work; Anna Lamp, my radiologist; and my anesthesiologist, Dr. Franchetti.

Here at long last I was able to conduct experiments in my special fields. At first I did not dare to put some of my ideas about corrective surgery into practice. Then one day a young couple arrived with a filly eight months old that they had vanned all the way from the eastern shore of Maryland. The filly was a beloved pet and they had taken her to veterinarian after veterinarian. All had said, "Destroy her. Nothing can be done."

The girl was crying as she explained: "We heard that you had some theory about how to correct this condition. You're our last hope. Can you do something?"

I had them walk the filly around. She hobbled badly, unable to put her right front foot to the ground. The X-rays showed exactly what I had suspected.

"I've never performed this operation, and as far as I know no one else has," I told them. "But your good little filly is in misery and unless I can correct the condition, she will have to be put down. If the operation succeeds, it will save hundreds—perhaps thousands—of horses in the future. Shall I try it?"

The couple conferred. "Go ahead," said the young man.

The mare was rolled into the surgery and I transected the inferior check ligament, lengthened it, carefully sutured all the adjacent tissue, then put the foot and leg in a plaster cast. I started operating at six in the evening and did not finish until midnight. Afterwards I could hardly sleep for worrying over the operation, and as soon as it was light the next morning I rushed down to examine the foot. If I was right, the results of the operation should have been immediately apparent. But the mare was still limping.

I took off the cast and worked the hoof back and forth by hand for a long time. Then I used an ace bandage, since I decided that the cast was too heavy and also prevented repeated manipulation of the leg, tendon, and hoof. The next day, I examined the mare again. Still no improvement. It could mean only one thing: I had been wrong. It was a cruel disappointment and I could not stand facing the hopeful young couple.

I was so discouraged that I did not bother to check the mare on the third morning. I saw Margaret coming up from the hospital, whistling merrily, and she waved to me as she went past. Although I knew it was hopeless, I asked her, "How's the filly coming alone?"

"Oh, fine," said Margaret casually. "She's standing with her heel on the ground. She seems all right."

"Why didn't you tell me!" I shouted, and rushed out to the hospital. The mare was standing normally for the first time in her life. I wandered around for the rest of the day in a happy trance as though I were high on drugs. The couple picked her up the following week. For several years they brought her back every six months so I could study the results of the operation and see how it affected the filly's movements.

I have published several papers on this and other techniques I developed for leg and foot ailments, and I hope that I have made a contribution to veterinary science that will be lasting.

A problem that has become increasingly important in the horse world is the use of drugs. When can they be considered legitimate? Some people feel that no horse should enter any competition if he has been drugged. Others point out that many otherwise excellent horses can be handled only if they have been given a tranquilizer to quiet them; otherwise they would have no use or purpose and would have to be put down. At a meeting held at the Devon Horse Show of 1978, it was proposed to pass a rule that no horse could be shown that had been given any kind of drug. This suggested ruling nearly produced a riot. Men who had come many miles to show their horses found themselves backed into a corner. The show's director was threatened with violence; emotions ran rampant and angry owners swore they'd not accept this decision quietly. It must be remembered that many of these men hoped to sell their horses for handsome profits, depending on how they did in the show. This ruling could cost them thousands of dollars.

Generally speaking, there are two different kinds of drugs used both at the racetrack and in the show ring. One is the phenylbutazone group, of which the best known is sold under the market name of butazolidin but is commonly known as "bute." "Bute" acts as an anti-inflammatory agent somewhat like aspirin. It reduces swelling and also pain but does not affect the horse's mental attitude. I believe its use is legitimate as long as the dosage is supervised and is not given secretly; for older horses with stiff joints such treatment is almost a necessity. Anabolic steroids are used by human athletes and can also be given to horses. They aid in the assimilation of food, stimulate the appetite, and settle the nerves. With them, the horse has several more years of useful life; without them, he may have to be destroyed. If I were a horse, I know which I'd prefer. It must be remembered that many people, especially older people, are dependent on certain drugs to make life bearable.

The other group consists largely of tranquilizers that affect the blood pressure, and in so doing, also affect the horse's reflexes. He cannot think clearly or make decisions. His whole personality changes. I have often seen horses under tranquilizers plunge headfirst into jumps, break their necks, or come crashing down on the track with broken legs. Vicious horses are given tranquilizers and then sold as being "gentle." Of course, when the drug wears off, the new owner finds the animal incorrigible. Tranquilized horses should never be entered in any competition.

On the other hand, if the use of "bute" were forbidden, I believe that 60 to 70 percent of the older horses could be neither raced nor shown. This seems a great waste. If the injection is given by a licensed veterinarian, openly, so that everyone knows it is being done, I consider it legitimate. I might add that there are a large number of drugs whose presence cannot be detected by any ordinary tests, and if the use of the standard phenylbutazones is stopped, it would be well-nigh impossible to prevent

215

owners from employing them. A few years ago in Florida when all drugs were forbidden, this is exactly what did occur, with serious results, as the people giving the injections had no idea what they were doing. Some of the horses suffered tremors and others even convulsed as a result.

When I was in veterinary school and said that I wanted to specialize in horses, I was told: "In a few years there'll be no more horses left. They're too expensive and difficult to keep and no one cares about them any more. The interest is in automobiles. Specialize in small animals." In any case, the idea of a woman being an equine practitioner was regarded as absurd. Women, I was often told, were not strong enough to handle horses and no one would entrust a valuable animal to a woman veterinarian. Today, there are more horses in America than there have ever been and I have never found that being a woman has handicapped me in any way. Being a veterinarian has not been an easy life. It is years since I've had a vacation; I am lucky when I get a full night's sleep. Without my family, I could not possibly have kept going. Yet it has been a rewarding life, never dull, always some new challenge, and always the feeling that I am doing something useful and important.

I am now contemplating building a second hospital near a racetrack. Not surprisingly, racehorses are constantly injuring their legs, and as I am daily gaining knowledge and experience, many of them are sent to me. This means vanning them a considerable distance; it would be much easier on the patients if I could treat them directly at the track. It would mean turning over at least some of my work to assistants, but I have already begun to train others in my methods.

Perhaps my most important current project is the technique of preventing painful nerve endings. When a nerve is severed, onion-shaped bodies called neuromas often grow on the proximal—closest to the body—cut ends. If this happens, pain begins again and the growth has to be cut away. This only results in another neuroma forming which, in turn, must also be removed. With new theories and methods developing, the nerve ending hopefully will remain inactive and not form a painful neuroma. If the new technique proves successful, it will be interesting as it can be used not only with animals but also with human beings and will alleviate a great deal of pain.

It seems that almost every week some new discoveries are being made in veterinary medicine which, in turn, suggest others, and so the science continues to grow. Already thousands of animals that a few years ago would have been destroyed as useless are now living happy, useful lives. An increasing number of the new discoveries either directly or indirectly affect the treatment of human beings. Sometimes I wonder if modern technology is not reaching a dead end. With the energy shortage, it may prove practical to use an increasing number of horses in farmwork. They reproduce themselves, raise their own food, and provide a natural fertilizer that in many respects is superior to any artificial product. Nothing gives me greater satisfaction than feeling that I am taking part in an increasingly important work, much of which is being recreated from old skills. And lastly, in case you did not guess, I love horses. It is wonderful to be able to spend your life doing something that you love.